TREATING CHRONICALLY MENTALLY ILL WOMEN

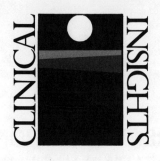

Judith H. Gold, M.D., F.R.C.P.(C)
Series Editor

TREATING CHRONICALLY MENTALLY ILL WOMEN

Edited by

LEONA L. BACHRACH, Ph.D.

Research Professor of Psychiatry, Maryland Psychiatric Research
Center, University of Maryland School of Medicine, Catonsville

CAROL C. NADELSON, M.D.

Professor and Vice Chairman, Department of Psychiatry,
Tufts University School of Medicine; Director of Training and
Education, Department of Psychiatry, Tufts–New England
Medical Center Hospitals

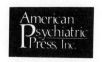

1400 K Street, N.W.
Washington, D.C. 20005

The paper used in this publication meets the minimum requirements of American National Standard for Information Sciences—Permanence of Paper for Printed Library Materials, ANSI Z39.48-1984.

Library of Congress Cataloging-in-Publication Data

Treating chronically mentally ill women / edited by Leona L. Bachrach, Carol C. Nadelson.
    p.   cm. — (Clinical insights)
    Proceedings of a symposium held at the 1986 American Psychiatric Association annual meeting in Washington, D.C.
    Includes bioliographies.
    ISBN-0-88048-144-7 (alk. paper)
    1. Mentally ill—Care—United States—Congresses.   2. Chronically ill—Care—United States—Congresses.   3. Women—Mental health services—United States—Congresses.   I. Bachrach, Leona L.
II. Nadelson, Carol C.   III. American Psychiatric Association. Meeting (139th : 1986 : Washington, D.C.)
IV. Series.
    [DNLM: 1. Chronic Disease—congresses.   2. Mental Disorders—therapy—congresses.   3. Women—psychology—congresses.
WM 400 T7835]
RC480.53.T74   1987
616.89′0088041—dc 19
DNLM/DLC
for Library of Congress   87-31830
                                                                          CIP

Contents

Contributors

Leona L. Bachrach, Ph.D.
Research Professor of Psychiatry, Maryland Psychiatric Research
Center, University of Maryland School of Medicine, Catonsville

Mona Bleiberg Bennett, M.D.
Deputy Commissioner, Massachusetts Department of Mental
Health, Boston

Jeanette Cochrane, B.A. Hon.
Mental Health Consultant, Clarke Institute of Psychiatry,
Toronto, Ontario

Jeffrey L. Geller, M.D., M.P.H.
Associate Professor of Psychiatry, University of Massachusetts
School of Medicine, Worcester

Paula Goering, R.N., Ph.D.
Senior Mental Health Consultant, Clarke Institute of Psychiatry,
Toronto, Ontario

Maryellen H. Handel, Ph.D.
Coordinator of Aftercare Services, Newton-Wellesley Hospital,
Newton, Massachusetts

William Lancee, M.Sc.
Research Coordinator, Clarke Institute of Psychiatry, Toronto,
Ontario

Dian Cox Leighton, B.S.
Director of the Family and Individual Reliance Project for the
Mental Health Association of Texas.

Marsha A. Martin, D.S.W.
Assistant Professor, Hunter College School of Social Work,
New York City

Mark R. Munetz, M.D.
Associate Professor of Psychiatry, University of Massachusetts
School of Medicine, Worcester

Carol C. Nadelson, M.D.
Professor and Vice Chairman, Department of Psychiatry,
Tufts University School of Medicine; Director of Training
and Education, Department of Psychiatry, Tufts–New England
Medical Center Hospitals

Doris T. Pearsall, Ph.D.
Director of Research and Evaluation, Massachusetts Department
of Mental Health, Boston

Harry Potasznik, M.A.
Research Assistant, Clarke Institute of Psychiatry, Toronto,
Ontario

Mary V. Seeman, M.D.
Psychiatrist-in-Chief, Mount Sinai Hospital, Toronto, Ontario;
Professor, Department of Psychiatry, University of Toronto,
Ontario

Donald Wasylenki, M.D., M.Sc.
Psychiatrist-in-Chief and Clinical Director, Whitby Psychiatric
Hospital, Whitby, Ontario

Introduction
to the Clinical Insights Series

*T*he Clinical Insights Series provides mental health–psychiatric clinicians with the most current information on a variety of topics of interest to them. These monographs are factual, up to date, and focused on areas of importance in daily professional interactions, whether in the private office, the outpatient clinic, or the inpatient unit. They are written for clinicians working in psychiatry and in other mental health professions.

Each year a number of monographs will be published dealing with all aspects of clinical practice. In addition, from time to time, a monograph may be revised and updated. Thus the Series will provide quick access to relevant and important areas of psychiatric practice. Some titles in the Series will be authored by a single expert; others will be edited by such an expert, who also will draw together other knowledgeable authors to produce a comprehensive overview of a topic.

Some of the monographs in the Clinical Insights Series will have their foundation in presentations at the annual meetings of the American Psychiatric Association. All will contain the most recent information on the subjects discussed. Within these compact volumes, theoretical and scientific data will be applied to clinical situations and case illustrations will be included, all with the practitioner in mind.

The special problems of the chronically mentally ill have aroused increasing concern over the past few years. *Treating Chronically Mentally Ill Women* is devoted to the treatment of women who are these patients and highlights their particular needs, which often are distinct from those of men. The Editors, Leona L. Bachrach, Ph.D., and Carol C. Nadelson, M.D., have carefully selected several authors to write about a number of relevant topics to illustrate the special problems of such women patients. Research data, clinical findings, and treatment modalities are discussed and clearly outlined in each chapter. Their thoughtful discussions of the points raised will be valuable for the clinician working with the chronically mentally ill.

Judith H. Gold, M.D., F.R.C.P.(C)
Series Editor,
Clinical Insights Series

Chapter 1

Chronically Mentally Ill Women: An Overview of Service Delivery Issues

LEONA L. BACHRACH, Ph.D.

Chapter 1

Chronically Mentally Ill Women: An Overview of Service Delivery Issues

The far-reaching differences between men and women have inspired curiosity, poetry, romance, and polemics for centuries, but they have only recently prompted scrutiny by social scientists. A key reason is that the social lives of men and women used to be more predictable; men typically behaved in certain ways and women in others. Gender differences in activities, goals, and longevity were taken for granted, being the persistent outcomes of quite predictable lives. At best, social statistics in this century reported data separately for men and women, but the fundamental scientific question "Why are there differences?" was not voiced. (1)

Recurrent themes in recent journal articles (2–9) and edited volumes (10–13) concerned with service planning for the chronically mentally ill are the changing demography and service requirements of this patient population; their demonstrated need for a full array of psychiatric, medical, social, vocational, and rehabilitative services, including asylum; the importance of integrating programmatic offerings for these individuals at both the administrative and direct-care levels; the effects of legal trends and decisions on these individuals' access to care; and the problems of assessing program outcomes in community-oriented service systems. A rich and sophisticated corpus of literature thus documents and underscores both the complexity of relevant service planning and the presence of numerous barriers to care for chronically mentally ill persons.

Yet, although the population of chronically mentally ill individuals consists of both women and men, relatively few contributions to the literature acknowledge, let alone discuss adequately, gender differences in patient careers or service requirements. Even fewer contributions focus on women's special circumstances (14). And although the number of writings addressing the needs of chronically mentally ill women appears to be on the increase (see Chapter 6), most of these pieces remain speculative and anecdotal. Many are found in the popular media instead of in professional sources (15). That professional writings on the chronically mentally ill are largely devoid of gender-specific questions is seriously at odds with the fact that issues of gender obviously are relevant for treatment planning. Life circumstances may differ dramatically for chronically mentally ill women and men, as is illustrated in the case of homeless individuals, many of whom suffer from chronic mental illnesses (16). Studies of residents in homeless shelters in Boston (17, 18) and in New York City (19) reveal that women exhibit significantly more severe psychopathology than men. At the Pine Street Inn, a renowned 350-bed "model" shelter in Boston, 90 percent of the women exhibit serious psychiatric problems, as contrasted with 40 percent of the men; and investigators conducting research at this facility conclude further that the psychiatric disabilities of homeless women are generally more complex and more severe than those of their male counterparts (17).

This chapter, an overview of the current literature on service delivery problems affecting the care of chronically mentally ill women, begins with a brief description of the population and underscores the depth and diversity of their service needs. Generally speaking, chronically mentally ill women are multiply disabled individuals. Like chronically mentally ill men, they suffer from the primary disabilities that characterize their illnesses, as well as from a multitude of derivative secondary disabilities, or "adverse personal reactions" (20), that endure even in the absence of primary symptoms (21). In addition, these women typically experience a variety of tertiary disabilities, or "social disablements" as described by Wing and Morris (20). Some of these social disablements are associated with their being chronic mental patients; others, however, appear to have more to do with their being women. Often these two kinds of social disablement interact to create serious deficits in the care of these women in today's psychiatric service systems.

In short, gender-determined considerations appear to be superimposed on more general problems associated with service delivery for chronic mental patients. The combination of these two circumstances—gender and chronicity—often produces serious problems in program planning for and treatment of chronically mentally ill women. This monograph has been prepared in recognition of the fact that such concerns must be addressed in any system of care that purports to be responsive to the needs of chronically mentally ill individuals.

Characteristics of the Population

The population of chronically mentally ill women consists of a variety of individuals. To think of them as a homogeneous group with uniform service requirements is to oversimplify their circumstances. Some within the population have resided in state mental hospitals, but others have not. Some appear to be faring well in the community, but others are clearly experiencing major difficulties. These women have been accorded a variety of diagnoses, and they possess differing treatment histories, functional levels, and prognoses. Accordingly, they require an extensive array of service structures and programmatic interventions.

The population of chronically mentally ill women in the United States has been profoundly affected by the policies, the practices, and the priorities that are associated with deinstitutionalization. Despite its promise of facilitating service delivery, deinstitutionalization has, almost paradoxically, served to complicate service planning by expanding the range of program needs within the base population of chronic mental patients (3, 4).

The outcomes of effecting deinstitutionalization plans have been varied. It is clear that, on the one hand, some chronically mentally ill women have benefited from the optimism and the innovative program offerings that are often part of deinstitutionalization. The quality of these women's lives has undoubtedly improved, as they have enrolled in community-based services that respond to their special needs. Some of these women have, in fact, gone on to become renowned writers and speakers who attempt to combat the stigma associated with chronic mental illness and who advocate ardently and articulately for better programs and more accessible entitlements for the chronically mentally ill (22, 23; see also Chapter 5).

At the same time, however, deinstitutionalization has had decidedly negative consequences for other chronically mentally ill women. Some members of the population, released from state mental hospitals without adequate treatment planning, have ended up in community settings with little more than a month's supply of medi-

5

cation. In a real sense, these are evicted women, and their existence is precarious. A few of them apparently adapt somehow to life outside the hospital. Others, however, return to the hospital, many of them repeatedly. And others, lacking community supports and the wherewithal to overcome barriers to their care, end up living on the streets, where they are at great risk for physical violence and abuse (15). These women are often "invisible" to psychiatric service providers (24), and aggressive outreach efforts are needed to engage them in the system of care (see Chapter 9).

Whether they are resident patients in state mental hospitals (see Chapter 10) or whether they reside in the community, chronically mentally ill women are often the victims of insensitive planning and inadequate services. Those who have been discharged from state mental hospitals are frequently at particularly high risk for disaffiliation and extrusion from the system of care. Even when they are actually placed appropriately in community-based facilities (when they are matched to residential and treatment settings consistent with their levels of functioning and prognoses), these women sometimes subsequently find themselves totally without homes when their living quarters are converted to other uses. Gentrification, which plays a role in the lives of many urban dwellers, is often particularly devastating for chronically mentally ill individuals and most especially so for the women among them (25).

Nor are those released from state mental hospitals the only chronically mentally ill women who have been adversely affected by deinstitutionalization policies and priorities. Even the lives of those who have never resided in state mental hospitals have been affected by the complex of events associated with deinstitutionalization. In its broadest sense deinstitutionalization discourages widespread utilization of state mental hospitals, often to such an extent that many women are denied admission to these facilities even when they are unable to secure desperately needed treatment or asylum elsewhere (7, 26, 27).

Many chronically mentally ill women also have been adversely affected by commitment procedures in various states. Although liberal commitment policies have the intent of protecting the civil rights of the chronically mentally ill, they sometimes, unfortunately, backfire. Legally barred from involuntary treatment and having no access to alternative residential facilities, many chronically mentally ill women become members of a special subgroup of the chronically mentally ill population who are homeless, have been homeless, or are at risk of becoming homeless (28–32; see also Chapter 9). Thus, chronically mentally ill women constitute a heterogeneous population with diverse needs for treatment and supportive services. But whatever their unique histories might be, these women tend to share certain circumstances. Very typically, they find themselves severely stigmatized by society (23, 31; see also Chapters 5 and 10). And poverty, disaffiliation, eviction, and physical abuse are constant threats to their survival (15, 25; see Chapters 6 and 9).

Program Needs

The service needs of chronically mentally ill women result from their illnesses, their multiple disabilities, and their special vulnerabilities. Every chronically mentally ill woman possesses a unique constellation of abilities and disabilities, and supports and deficiencies, that together determine her specific treatment requirements. Nevertheless, it is probably accurate to generalize that, for virtually all of these women, there is a need for access to high-quality psychiatric care. The psychiatric service system thus must make available to chronically mentally ill women a variety of individually prescribed psychotherapeutic interventions, including carefully monitored psychotropic medications.

This need for psychiatric services is generally supplemented by a need for housing. That appropriate and affordable residential opportunities constitute a basic program dimension for chronically mentally ill individuals is an established aspect of service planning (2). The array of residences offered must be an extensive one, including both temporary and permanent kinds of accommodations. Some chronically mentally ill women require housing that affords them temporary refuge and asylum in the face of precipitate crisis. Other women need somewhat longer, but still short-term, temporary housing for those times when their permanent residences fail to serve their current needs. Still other women require placement in long-term residential facilities, perhaps for the rest of their lives.

However, it must be stressed that, although chronically mentally ill women in this era of deinstitutionalization must be provided with access to appropriate residences, housing by itself is only one of several major dimensions in service planning for this population (16, 18). It is essential that residential services be supplemented by access to a full complement of medical, social, vocational, rehabilitative, and recreational services. For some chronically mentally ill women, it may even be necessary to arrange for the provision of basic life necessities: food, clothing, and primary health care (see Chapters 7, 8, and 9).

In addition, these basic structural program offerings for chronically mentally ill women, as for their male counterparts, must be provided in a service milieu that is best described as one that enhances continuity of care (33; see Chapter 8). The notion of continuity of care is an outgrowth of post-World War II health planning initiatives. Properly understood, it promotes comprehensive, accessible, individualized, and culturally relevant services to patients over a long period of time, in a predictably supportive and human manner.

Service Delivery Issues

Despite the fact that chronically mentally ill women generally require comprehensive services and continuity in their care, a variety of factors tend to inhibit their access to relevant treatment programs. In addition to those circumstances that affect the care of chronically mentally ill individuals of both sexes, certain special issues are barriers to the appropriate care of chronically mentally ill women in today's psychiatric service systems. These may be classified into three broad categories: minimization of individual differences, absence of relevant research, and failure to implement established research findings.

Minimization of Individual Differences

Stereotyped program planning for chronically mentally ill women tends to minimize differences within the population and to lump these individuals together as if they have homogeneous service needs. Often, such stereotypes have their origins in prevailing sex-role expectations for women. Primary care physicians are known in general to have biased preconceptions of women's health care needs (34), and it would be surprising if psychiatrists and other mental health professionals did not share in such stereotyped ideas.

Rehabilitative skills training programs for chronically mentally ill women provide a specific example. Such programs often encourage these patients to assume relatively dependent roles and to be either unemployed or employed in such domestic pursuits as housecleaning and babysitting (15, 35; see also Chapter 6), even though work is an important factor in the lives of psychiatrically disabled women (see Chapter 4). By contrast, programs for men tend to focus on their eventual readiness for competitive employment (15, 35).

Strasser (36) describes gender-related role expectations in a soup kitchen and drop-in center for homeless individuals, many of whom are chronically mentally ill:

> No services were asked from women, although cooperation with procedures was expected . . . [Men] were often expected to contribute some service as well as to follow routine. Women not only entered for meals ahead of all men, sick, injured, or well, but occasionally women who arrived late for meals were served, while men would be turned away if late. The service was regarded . . . as "lady's privilege."

There is clearly an assumption here that the well-being of women requires fewer challenges than that of men—an assumption that is consistent with Wagner and associates' (37) observation that "women in American society are generally expected to be less capable than men, particularly in situations involving some sort of task performance." The implications of holding such stereotypes in service planning for chronically mentally ill women should be obvious. They may reinforce female patients' helplessness rather than encourage their independence, a practice that might well be clinically inappropriate (38, 39). Although such stereotyped planning is now being challenged in the literature, it continues, in biased fashion, to shape the dimensions of service offerings for chronically mentally ill women today (38, 40).

Absence of Relevant Research

A second issue, closely related to the problem of stereotyped planning, concerns the general absence of relevant research on the service needs of chronically mentally ill women. If planners already "know" what women require, they may neglect to investigate gender-specific program needs. Thus, even when chronically mentally ill women have been provided with appropriately individualized clinical assessments, there is often a limited body of knowledge on which to base gender-relevant program decisions (see Chapter 3).

The current literature, in fact, points to a variety of program

9

planning concerns that might profit from more extensive gender-focused research. In some of these areas, studies have already been conducted, but supplemental validating investigations are needed (see Chapter 6). For example, additional research is required to sort out the correlates of gender-specific neurological side effects of psychotropic agents (5, 41–43; see also Chapter 2). Hauser (44) reviews risks inherent in the use of antidepressants, antipsychotics, anxiolytics, and lithium by pregnant women, a matter of timely concern (46–49) in view of reported increases in fertility within the chronically mentally ill female population (50, 51).

Also needed is research documenting the demographic correlates of chronic mental illness among women. Age and ethnicity are variables that apparently interact with gender to create unique service needs among chronically mentally ill women. For example, Dworkin and Adams (48) report that the interaction of gender and ethnicity may have a profound effect on both diagnosis and treatment planning for chronically mentally ill individuals. Similarly, problems specific to treating geriatric chronic mental patients may largely be considered women's problems because of the excess of elderly females in the population (52). Black and his colleagues (53) report that the excess age-specific mortality rates among patients discharged from state mental hospitals are particularly marked for women. Additional studies are needed to investigate the correlates of this phenomenon.

Similarly, more research is needed to assess the correlates of homelessness among chronically mentally ill women. It is not at all clear why, as noted previously, homeless women tend to have more serious psychiatric problems than homeless men. Nor is it clear what circumstances propel many of these women into jails and other correctional facilities (54). Indeed, the psychiatric needs of women in prisons require much more investigation (55). Those within the prison population who also suffer from chronic mental illnesses undoubtedly constitute an overwhelmingly underserved group of individuals.

In the area of service delivery, research is needed to determine the ways in which gatekeeping practices differentially affect the access of chronically mentally ill women to needed psychiatric services and thus shape their patient careers (see Chapter 8). Shelters serving homeless women, unlike those for homeless men, frequently exclude or extrude individuals who are drunk, physically disabled,

10

or suspected of using hard drugs (56). Moreover, women living in such shelters, unlike men, may systematically be "rotated" out of them—a situation described in this way by a nun working in a New York City shelter:

> You see, we only have beds here for twelve women and we let twelve more women sleep sitting up in chairs. But there are thousands of women out there—thousands who have no place to live. So many ladies come here for shelter that we can only let them stay for four days before we send them back out on the streets. We call it "rotation." Four days in, three days out. It's horrible, but we don't have much choice. (57)

Clearly, investigations into the outcomes of such practices are indicated. Kates (57) reports the death of one schizophrenic homeless woman while she was living on the streets during such a rotation.

To recapitulate, then, the development of appropriate and relevant programs for chronically mentally ill women is at times hampered by the practice of subordinating their individual requirements to stereotyped and global notions of women's needs. This difficulty is compounded by a general paucity of research findings on important topics that might indicate new directions in service planning for members of this patient population.

Failure to Implement Research Findings

A third issue limiting the access of chronically mentally ill women to needed services is the lag that often develops between what researchers know and what service agencies do. Even when appropriate directions in program development have been established, it may take considerable time before they are implemented in the real world of service delivery (see Chapter 6).

This situation is illustrated in the case of chronically mentally ill women who are pregnant. It is widely agreed that such women have special service requirements that must be met and that their need for adequate psychiatric and supportive care is profound. However, far from responding to their extraordinary program requirements, psychiatric service systems may actually bar pregnant women's access to the most basic of services, such as housing (56). Pregnant women are, in fact, sometimes extruded from the residential facilities in which they have been placed; and they may experience great difficulties in securing substitute housing, as this poignant and disturbing excerpt from a case history reported by Kates (57) indicates:

> The other women worried about Gwendolyn alone on the [park] bench. They knew what Gwendolyn refused to admit. She was pregnant. They begged local churches to take her in. They explained why they were so concerned. But no one offered Gwendolyn any other place to live ... Gwendolyn gave birth on the bench outside the locked building where she had once lived.

Unfortunately, there are probably many Gwendolyns in many communities in the United States. The plight of these women often reflects a more general inability on the part of the psychiatric service system to respond sensitively to the multiplicity of special service needs that chronically mentally ill women may experience.

Conclusions

Subsequent chapters in this monograph provide more detailed discussion of the uniqueness of the service requirements of chronically mentally ill women and of the ways in which service systems often overlook or deny their special needs. The foregoing discussion has introduced the subject of this monograph by documenting the fact that general barriers to care among the chronically mentally ill— that is, barriers that are not gender specific—are often exacerbated by inadequate attention to gender-related issues (58, 59). Available services often appear at best to be irrelevant to the special requirements of chronically mentally ill women. At worst they may be frankly discriminatory. Thus, as Dworkin and Adams (48) point out, "gender remains a critical variable" in the study of chronic mental illness.

Within the larger population of chronically mentally ill individuals there are certain subpopulations whose special service needs are generally known to be overlooked in traditional or established programs (60, 61). Dually diagnosed individuals, whether their psychiatric illnesses coexist with developmental disabilities or with substance abuse problems, often fit that description. The elderly chronically mentally ill constitute another such subpopulation (61).

One may conclude that chronically mentally ill women to some extent share extraordinary barriers to care with these other underserved subpopulations. Like them, chronically mentally ill women often appear to be excessively stigmatized. For chronically mentally ill women, as for members of these other subpopulations, programmatic irrelevance may result from stereotyped planning, from the system's failure to identify special service requirements, and from a general absence of appropriate service-related research. Further irrelevance may ensue when the service system fails to implement new programmatic solutions even though their efficacy has been documented by research.

Women currently constitute nearly two-thirds of the population of chronically mentally ill individuals in the United States (62). It is essential that the vestiges of stereotyped thinking about their service requirements be eliminated; that discriminatory practices, whether they are intended or not, be removed; and that planning within the system of care be adapted to meet the special needs of this service population.

References

1. Verbrugge LM: Gender and health: an update on hypotheses and evidence. J Health Soc Behav 26:156–182, 1985
2. Bachrach LL: Planning services for chronically mentally ill patients. Bull Menninger Clin 47:163–188, 1983
3. Bachrach LL: Asylum and chronically ill psychiatric patients. Am J Psychiatry 141:975–978, 1984
4. Bachrach LL: The young adult chronic psychiatric patient in an era of deinstitutionalization. Am J Public Health 74:382–384, 1984
5. Braun P, Kochansky G, Shapiro R, et al: Overview: deinstitutionalization of psychiatric patients: a critical review of outcome studies. Am J Psychiatry 138:736–749, 1981
6. Mollica RF: From asylum to community: the threatened disintegration of public psychiatry. N Engl J Med 308:367–373, 1983
7. Pepper B, Ryglewicz H: Testimony for the neglected: the mentally ill in the post-deinstitutionalization age. Am J Orthopsychiatry 52:388–391, 1982
8. Santiago JM, McCall-Perez F, Bachrach LL: Integrated services for chronic mental patients: theoretical perspective and experimental results. Gen Hosp Psychiatry 7:309–315, 1985

9. Freedman RI, Moran A: Wanderers in a promised land: the chronically mentally ill and deinstitutionalization. Care 22 (Suppl): S1-S60, 1984
10. Stein LI, Test MA (eds): Alternatives to Mental Hospital Treatment. New York, Plenum, 1978
11. Talbott JA (ed): The Chronic Mental Patient: Problems, Solutions, and Recommendations for a Public Policy. Washington, DC, American Psychiatric Association, 1978
12. Talbott JA (ed): The Chronic Mentally Ill: Treatment, Programs, Systems. New York, Human Sciences Press, 1981
13. Talbott, JA (ed): The Chronic Mental Patient: Five Years Later. Orlando, FL, Grune & Stratton, 1984
14. Geller JL: Women's accounts of psychiatric illness and institutionalization. Hosp Community Psychiatry 36:1056-1062, 1985
15. Bachrach LL: Deinstitutionalization and women: assessing the consequences of public policy. Am Psychol 39:1171-1177, 1984
16. Lamb HR (ed): The Homeless Mentally Ill. Washington, DC, American Psychiatric Association, 1984
17. Lenehan GP, McInnes BN, O'Donnell D, et al: A nurses' clinic for the homeless. Am J Nursing 1237-1240, 1985
18. McGerigle P, Lauriat AS: More Than Shelter: A Community Response to Homelessness. Boston, United Planning Corporation and Massachusetts Association for Mental Health, 1983
19. Crystal S: Homeless men and women: the gender gap. Urban and Social Change Review 17(Summer):2-6, 1984
20. Wing JK, Morris B. Clinical basis of rehabilitation, in Handbook of Psychiatric Rehabilitation Practice. Edited by Wing JK, Morris B. London, Oxford University Press, 1981, pp 3-16
21. Shepherd G: Institutional Care and Rehabilitation. London, Longman, 1984
22. Lovejoy M: Recovery from schizophrenia: a personal odyssey. Hosp Community Psychiatry 35:809-812, 1984
23. Bache-Snyder K: Esso Leete battles stigma of mental illness. Longmont (Colorado) Times-Call, 6 October 1985, p 5B
24. Teltsch K: A haven for Boston's "invisible women." New York Times, 31 March 1986, p B7
25. Harrington M: The New American Poverty. New York, Holt, Rinehart & Winston, 1984
26. Dionne EJ: Mental patient cutbacks planned. New York Times, 8 December 1978, p B3

27. Sullivan R: Hospital forced to oust patients with psychoses. New York Times, 8 November 1979, p. A1
28. Allen A: Who killed Rebecca Smith? Foundation News 24: 13–16, 1982
29. Carmody D: The tangled life and mind of Judy, whose home is the street. New York Times, 17 December 1984, pp B1, B10
30. Herman R: One of the city's homeless goes home—in death. New York Times, 27 October 1981, p B3
31. McKay P: My home is a lonely bed in a dreary D.C. shelter. Washington Post, 16 February 1986, pp C1, C3
32. Bachrach LL: Interpreting research on the homeless mentally ill. Some caveats. Hosp Community Psychiatry 35:914–917, 1984
33. Bachrach LL: Continuity of care for chronic mental patients: a conceptual analysis. Am J Psychiatry 138:1449–1456, 1981
34. Bernstein B, Kane R: Physicians' attitudes toward female patients. Med Care 19:600–608, 1981
35. Keskiner A, Zalcman MH, Rupert EH: Advantages of being female in psychiatric rehabilitation. Arch Gen Psychiatry 28: 689–692, 1973
36. Strasser J: Urban transient women. Am J Nursing 2078–2079, 1978
37. Wagner DG, Ford RS, Ford TW: Can gender inequalities be reduced? American Sociological Review 51:47–61, 1986
38. Women's Task Force: For Better or Worse? Women and the Mental Health System. Lansing, Michigan Department of Mental Health, April 1982
39. Houghton J: On personal experience: before and after mental illness, in Attitudes Toward the Mentally Ill: Research Perspectives. Edited by Rabkin JG, Gelb L, Lazar JB. Rockville, MD, National Institute of Mental Health, 1980, pp 7–14
40. Test MA, Berlin SB: Issues of special concern to chronically mentally ill women. Professional Psychology 12:136–145, 1981
41. Seeman MV: Schizophrenic men and women require different treatment programs. Journal of Psychiatric Treatment and Evaluation 5:143–148, 1983
42. Seeman MV: Gender differences in schizophrenia. Can J Psychiatry 27:107–112, 1982
43. Smith JM, Dunn DD: Sex differences in the prevalence of severe tardive dyskinesia. Am J Psychiatry 136:1080–1083, 1979

44. Hauser LA: Pregnancy and psychiatric drugs. Hosp Community Psychiatry 36:817–818, 1985
45. Mogul KM: Psychological considerations in the use of psychotropic drugs with women patients. Hosp Community Psychiatry 36:1080–1085, 1985
46. Nurnberg H, Prudic J: Guidelines for treatment of psychosis during pregnancy. Hosp Community Psychiatry 35:67–71, 1984
47. Remick RA, Maurice WL: ECT in pregnancy (letter). Am J Psychiatry 135:761–762, 1978
48. Dworkin RJ, Adams GL: Pharmacotherapy of the chronic patient: gender and diagnostic factors. Community Mental Health J 20:253–261, 1984
49. Nurnberg HG: Treatment of mania in the last six months of pregnancy. Hosp Community Psychiatry 31:122–126, 1980
50. Pepper B, Ryglewicz H: Treating the young adult chronic patient: an update, in Advances in Treating the Young Adult Chronic Patient. (New Directions for Mental Health Services no. 21). San Francisco, Jossey-Bass, 1984
51. Test MA, Knoedler W, Allness DJ, et al: Characteristics of young adults with schizophrenic disorders treated in the community. Hosp Community Psychiatry 36:853–858, 1985
52. Cicchinelli LF, Bell JC, Dittmar ND, et al: Factors Influencing the Deinstitutionalization of the Mentally Ill: A Review and Analysis. Denver, Denver Research Institute, 1981
53. Black DW, Warrack G, Winokur G: Excess mortality among psychiatric patients. JAMA 253:58–61, 1985
54. Lamb HR, Grant RW: Mentally ill women in a county jail. Arch Gen Psychiatry 40:363–368, 1983
55. Goldstein N: Women in prison: a neglected population. Hosp Community Psychiatry 36:1027, 1985
56. Baxter E, Hopper K: The new mendicancy: homeless in New York City. Am J Orthopsychiatry 52:393, 408, 1982
57. Kates B: The Murder of a Shopping Bag Lady. San Diego, Harcourt Brace Jovanovich, 1985
58. Hauser P, Finkelberg F, Pollack BN, et al: Risk and protective factors in schizophrenia: clinical and social implications. Modern Medicine of Canada 40:579–584, 1985
59. Hauser P, Seeman MV: Schizophrenia in males vs. females. Medical Aspects of Human Sexuality 19:109–119, 1985

60. President's Commission on Mental Health: Report to the President. Washington, DC, U.S. Government Printing Office, 1978
61. Bachrach LL: The context of care for the chronic mental patient with substance abuse problems. Psychiatric Q 58:3–14, 1986/ 1987
62. Asbaugh JW, Leaf PJ, Manderscheid RW, et al: Estimates of the size and selected characteristics of the adult chronically mentally ill population living in U.S. households. Research in Community and Mental Health 3:3–24, 1983

Chapter 2

Schizophrenia in Women and Men

MARY V. SEEMAN, M.D.

Chapter 2

Schizophrenia in Women and Men

Dr. Seeman succinctly delineates gender differences in schizophrenia, including age of onset and neuroleptic response. She considers hypotheses and treatment implications for these data.

Onset age and neuroleptic response are two of many factors predictive of chronicity in schizophrenia. The earlier the age of onset, the more severe the illness usually is, and the greater the likelihood that it will take a chronic course (1). With respect to neuroleptic response, those individuals whose form of illness responds best to neuroleptic drugs and who are least sensitive to the adverse side effects of these drugs usually display a more remitting, less chronic course of illness (2).

Both these factors, onset age and neuroleptic response, differ between men and women.

Onset Age

The earlier the onset, the worse the prognosis. Most investigators, although not all, agree that onset in women is several years later than in men (3–6). This earlier onset for men is certainly true where broad definitions of schizophrenia are used. "Narrow" diagnoses that exclude prominent affective symptoms from the schizophrenic sample tend to narrow the onset-age discrepancy (6).

If we assume that onset-age differences between men and women do exist in an illness that we agree to call schizophrenia, however it is diagnosed, what reasons might there be for the discrepancy?

There may be several, depending on how we conceptualized this illness and its underlying causes and triggering factors.

If schizophrenia is a hyperdopaminergic illness, we know that female hormones, estrogens, are antidopaminergic and female elevation of estrogens in puberty may delay schizophrenia onset (7).

21

If schizophrenia is an illness lateralized to one or the other brain hemisphere, then women's more bilateral representation of brain functions may be protective and delay the illness (7).

If the schizophrenia threshold is lowered by brain trauma, it is known that male infants suffer more than female infants from perinatal brain injury and also from head trauma during childhood and adolescence (7).

If schizophrenia is associated with viral infection, males and females have different immune systems. The thymus involutes in adolescence earlier in males than in females and may render males relatively immunodeficient (7).

If certain triggers such as alcohol and drug abuse or familial demand and criticism bring schizophrenia illness forward in time, then, again, it is generally believed that male adolescents are disproportionally exposed to these potential precipitants (7).

If social supports are important protective factors, then it is also probably true that young women have more close friends than do young men and are more affectively linked with friends, relatives, and help-givers. It may be that certain early indications of the schizophrenic process, such as social withdrawal, lack of ambition, or unpredictable aggressiveness, are more easily tolerated in women than in men and are less likely to cause the loss of friends or the support of families (8).

Many other biological, psychological, or social role differences between men and women may account for onset-age differences, although it must be remembered that these differences have been reported since the time of Kraepelin and have been noted all over the world. In other words, they must be relatively immutable phenomena that do not depend on local or cultural variations.

Neuroleptic Response

The older literature on the time spent hospitalized for schizophrenia shows longer lengths of stay for women. The newer literature shows shorter lengths of stay for women (9). This change may have to do with women's longer life span in the era before the 1950s, when hospitalization for schizophrenia meant staying in the hospital until the time of death. It may also have to do with the introduction of neuroleptics.

Are women more responsive to the beneficial effects of neuroleptics than men? There is some evidence that they are. Kolakowska and co-workers have reported on the quality of neuroleptic response of 77 schizophrenic patients meeting Research Diagnostic Criteria (RDC), 28 women and 49 men. Response was judged by symptom alleviation during a current exacerbation of illness. Seventy-five percent were under the age of 40. Using a response classification developed in an earlier study, this research group found that their responders consisted of a significantly high proportion of female subjects (10).

Young and Meltzer (11) reported on neuroleptic response during acute psychosis of 61 schizophrenic patients diagnosed by the *Diagnostic and Statistical Manual of Mental Disorders (Second Edition)* criteria (12). Thirty-one improved on placebo or low-dose neuroleptics (no higher than 200 mg chlorpromazine [CPZ] equivalents per day) and 30 later improved on high-dose neuroleptics (800 mg or more of CPZ equivalents per day). There was a significant gender difference between the low-dose versus high-dose improvement groups. Seventy percent of the men who improved were in the high-dose group, whereas 61 percent of the women who improved were in the placebo or low-dose group. There were no age differences between the low- and high-dose groups. The overall mean age was 27 years. Women seemed to require lower doses than men to achieve control of acute symptoms. Women also seem to require—at least in their younger years—a lower maintenance dose to prevent psychotic relapse. After age 40 their maintenance doses may, however, exceed those of men. I surveyed 101 outpatient schizophrenic patients diagnosed by RDC criteria, 43 women and 58 men. Male and female mean CPZ equivalent doses were the same, but younger women (ages 20–39) were maintained at lower doses than in a similar age group. After age 40, women required higher doses than men to prevent psychotic recurrence (13).

Dworkin and Adams (14) studied 1,752 (age range, 17–91 years; mean, 47 years) ambulatory patients who were treated in community mental health centers. Of these, 990 were diagnosed as schizophrenic, by criteria that were unspecified. Four hundred ninety-nine subjects were men; 491 were women. Males were significantly younger than females. Men received significantly higher doses of antipsychotics, but this effect was eliminated by including age in the analysis, as age showed an inverse relationship to dose in

23

the group as a whole. Separate relationships among age, sex, and class were not reported.

Women appear to do better in the long run, although, again, it looks as if the diagnostic criteria for schizophrenia are important (15). Studies using narrowly defined criteria are not as likely to show female advantage as those based on broad definitions (16). A differential susceptibility to neuroleptics is suggested by the fact that the superior outcome for women has become apparent only in the postneuroleptic era. Watt and co-workers (17) followed 121 schizophrenics (Present State Examination) for five years. There were 61 male and 60 female subjects, ranging in age from 17 to 60 years. Forty-eight of the patients were first admissions. Of this first-admission group, the clinical outcome was significantly worse for the men. Thirty-two percent of the women (compared with 15 percent of the men) had only one episode with no subsequent impairment. Approximately equivalent percentages of men and women had more than one episode with minimal impairment. However, 46 percent of the men (compared with 18 percent of the women) had impairment increasing with each of several episodes, with no return to normality.

Considering the whole group (first and subsequent admissions), the outcome was again worse for the men. Thirty-five percent of the men and 62 percent of the women were in the good-outcome groups, while 58 percent of the men and only 26 percent of the women were in the most severely affected group. Significantly more women than men remained out of the hospital during the follow-up period. Watt and colleagues noted that the advantage for female patients found in this study was not seen in a five-year follow-up of first-admission schizophrenic patients at the same hospital in an earlier time period (17).

Long-term outcome studies may actually mask the apparent short-term advantage for women because the final follow-up is done at a time when the female subjects are over 40 or into their menopause.

Why should the age of the female subjects matter?

It matters if the prevailing theory is true: that the reason why neuroleptics work better in women is because they are "helped along" by female hormones; that is, estrogens (3, 18).

Estrogens are dopamine antagonists in experimental animals. Clinically, it appears that psychotic symptoms in schizophrenia are exaggerated premenstrually and especially postpartum, when estrogen levels fall (7). Schizophrenic women are relatively symptom free during pregnancy, when levels are high (7). Symptoms are often exacerbated at menopause, when estrogen levels are falling (7). At this stage, women seem to need higher doses of neuroleptics than men, as if the withdrawal of estrogens had caused a rebound effect on symptoms (13). This same mechanism is thought to operate in the phenomenon of menopausal tardive dyskinesia, with the withdrawal of estrogens again acting like a withdrawal of neuroleptics (since the two are synergistic) and producing a "withdrawal dyskinesia" (19).

Different vulnerabilities of men and women to acute and subacute extrapyramidal symptoms also are compatible with this theory. Men are more susceptible to the acute dystonias, which are caused by the abrupt disruption of the dopamine-acetylcholine balance by the sudden introduction of dopamine blockers. In women, whose dopamine receptors are already somewhat blocked by cyclic estrogens, the suddenness of neuroleptic action is tempered (20).

Women are, however, more prone than men to the later extrapyramidal effects of cogwheeling, tremor, akithesia, and akinesia. This may be because estrogens and neuroleptics together cause a cumulatively stronger dopaminergic blockade than that caused by neuroleptics alone (20).

There are, of course, other reasons why the effective neuroleptic dose may vary between men and women. There are indications that women are more likely to continue with their prescribed dose, whether they are uncomfortable because of side-effects or not (21). They are proportionately smaller in size and may not require as high a dose for that reason. In addition, they have proportionally more lipid stores, and neuroleptics accumulate in adipose tissue. This may be the reason why, after stopping neuroleptics, women may continue longer than men to be free of relapse and also to suffer side-effects (22).

Treatment Implications

What are the treatment implications of these observations? How can we help prevent chronicity in both sexes by fending off schizophrenia onset as long as possible and ensuring the judicious (not too high and not too low) dose of neuroleptics?

We need to prevent birth injury and head trauma, enhance the immune system (perhaps by psychological means), and ensure good nutrition in adolescence, especially in young women so that puberty is not delayed. We need to avoid any known or suspected triggers to schizophrenia onset, especially in families thought to be at genetic risk. We also need to advocate for close social supports and a responsive medical-psychosocial system of care.

Once schizophrenia has begun, we need to be careful about our neuroleptic doses. In women, if doses are raised beyond a certain individual threshold, menstrual periods cease and the natural protection of estrogens may be eliminated (18). We need to keep doses low. We may need to give none or less at certain times of the month when estrogen levels are relatively high. At menopause, schizophrenia may need to be added to the list of possible indications for estrogen supplementation.

Although these measures may or may not help protect against chronicity, they should be tried on an experimental basis, with proper precautions, to confirm whether they can enhance the quality of life of the schizophrenic population. The schizophrenic patient's life is a difficult one, but some individuals fare better with this illness than others. In general, we know women fare better. Through research based on that observation, we may be able to help both women and men.

References

1. Zigler E, Levine J: Age on first hospitalization of schizophrenics: a developmental approach. J Abnorm Psychol 96: 458–467, 1981
2. Seeman MV: Clinical and demographic correlates of neuroleptic response. Can J Psychiatry 30:243–245, 1985
3. Bellodi L, Morabito A, Macciardi F, et al: Analytic considerations about observed distribution of age of onset in schizophrenia. Neuropsychobiology 8:93–101, 1982
4. Lewine RRJ: Sex differences in age of symptom onset and first hospitalization in schizophrenia. Am J Orthopsychiatry 50: 316–222, 1980
5. Loranger AW: Sex differences in age at onset of schizophrenia. Arch Gen Psychiatry 41:157–161, 1984
6. Leventhal DB, Schuckit JR, Rothstein H: Gender differences in schizophrenia. J Nerv Ment Dis 172:464–467, 1984

7. Seeman MV: Sex and schizophrenia. Can J Psychiatry 30: 313–315, 1985
8. Busfield J: Gender and mental illness. Int J Mental Health 11:46–66, 1982
9. Seeman MV: Current outcome in schizophrenia: women vs. men. Acta Psychiatr Scand 73:609–617, 1986
10. Kolakowska T, Williams AO, Ardern M, et al: Schizophrenia with good and poor outcome. I. Early clinical features, response to neuroleptics and signs of organic dysfunction. Br J Psychiatry 146:229–246, 1985
11. Young MA, Meltzer HY: The relationship of demographic, clinical, and outcome variables to neuroleptic treatment requirements. Schizophrenia Bull 6:88–101, 1980
12. American Psychiatric Association. Diagnostic and Statistical Manual of Mental Disorders (Second Edition). Washington, DC, American Psychiatric Association, 1968
13. Seeman MV: Interaction of sex, age, and neuroleptic dose. Compr Psychiatry 24:125–128, 1983
14. Dworkin RJ, Adams GL: Pharmacotherapy of the chronic patient: gender and diagnostic factors. Community Ment Health J 20:253–261, 1984
15. Salokongas RKR: Prognostic implications of the sex of schizophrenic patients. Br J Psychiatry 142:145–151, 1983
16. MacMillan JF, Crow TJ, Johnson AL, et al: The Northwick Park study of first episodes of schizophrenia. III. Short-term outcome in trial entrants and trial eligible patients. Br J Psychiatry 148:128–133, 1986
17. Watt DC, Katz K, Shepherd M: The natural history of schizophrenia: a 5-year prospective follow-up of a representative sample of schizophrenics by means of a standardized clinical and social assessment. Psychol Med 13:663–670, 1983
18. Seeman MV: Gender and the onset of schizophrenia: neurohumoral influences. Psychiatr J Univ Ottawa 6:136–138, 1981
19. Seeman MV: Schizophrenic men and women require different treatment programs. Journal of Psychiatric Treatment and Evaluation 5:143–148, 1983
20. Seeman MV: Gender differences in schizophrenia. Can J Psychiatry 27:107–112, 1982

21. Kessler RC, Brown RL, Broman CL: Sex differences in psychiatric help-seeking: evidence from four large scale surveys. J Health Soc Behav 22:49–64, 1981
22. Lehmann HE, Ban IA: Sex differences in long-term adverse effects of phenothiazines, in Phenothiazines and Structurally Related Drugs. Edited by Forrest IS, Carr CJ, Usdin E. New York, Raven Press, 1974

Chapter 3

Behavioral Differences Between Female and Male Hospitalized Chronically Mentally Ill Patients

MONA BLEIBERG BENNETT, M.D.
MARYELLEN H. HANDEL, Ph.D.
DORIS T. PEARSALL, Ph.D.

Chapter 3

Behavioral Differences Between Female and Male Hospitalized Chronically Mentally Ill Patients

The authors of this chapter report on a study of almost 2,000 hospitalized male and female chronic mental patients. They found significant differences between the groups with regard to behavior and treatment. The males were more physically and sexually threatening and more assaultive than the females. The females frequently made suicide attempts and threats, abused themselves physically, manifested sleep disturbances, were more verbally abusive, had temper tantrums, and publically disrobed. They were more frequently chemically restrained than were the men. These data confirm other reports and emphasize the need to acknowledge, understand, and plan specific programs that address these gender differences.

While there is a sizable body of literature on various aspects of gender influences in psychotherapy, there is little that focuses on the how gender affects the ways that signs and symptoms are expressed or how it affects the care of hospitalized chronically mentally ill patients. This general lack of attention to gender differences in chronic mental illness is cited by several authors (1–4). Test and Berlin (3), for example, write that there "appears to be a pervasive lack of research, thought, or sensitivity to gender-related issues" as they relate to members of the chronically mentally ill population. Furthermore, according to these authors, clinicians often fail to respond to chronically mentally ill individuals as sex-differentiated persons.

Gender-related demographic differences among those who have been diagnosed with schizophrenia have, however, been reported. It has been noted, for example, that age at first hospitalization is significantly lower for men than for women and that men are significantly overrepresented among hospitalized young adult schizophrenics (4–9). Studies also suggest that age at onset of illness is lower for men (8). Both biological (5, 9) and social factors (6) have been proposed to explain these findings.

Women, on the other hand, are disproportionately overrepresented on hospital wards in middle and later life (3). This circumstance appears to be related not only to the relatively greater longevity of women but also to a higher incidence of affective disorder among women (5) and to the relatively delayed onset of both affective disorder and schizophrenia.

Whatever the relative contributions of biological and environmental factors to these circumstances may be, one might well expect that they would have major implications for ego development and character formation, as well as for social, educational, and vocational experiences. These events affect both the expression of illness among chronic mental patients and approaches for their care, treatment, and rehabilitation. It is precisely because of such considerations that Seeman (10) argues that "schizophrenic men and women require different treatment programs."

This chapter presents data that should stimulate further research on both the role of gender differences in the expression of chronic mental illness and the design of programs appropriate to the care of this very ill patient population. The study reported here analyzes findings from a large data set collected between July 1, 1982, and June 30, 1983. The study population includes 1,898 patients hospitalized in the seven state mental hospitals in Massachusetts. Although largely an exploratory effort, this study is unique in establishing the existence of behavioral differences and differential treatment needs and interventions, according to gender, within a large and unsampled statewide state hospital inpatient population.

Methodology

The larger study from which the data reported here are derived was designed by the Massachusetts Department of Mental Health to assess all inpatients' clinical needs so that management issues concerning appropriateness of care and plans for additional services might be addressed. A modified version of the New York State level-of-care instrument, developed in 1975 by the New York State Department of Mental Hygiene, was used toward these ends. Information was gathered on a wide variety of events, including sociodemographic variables, sensory impairment, somatic and psychogenic conditions and their relationship to functioning, skill levels in activities of daily living, behavioral manifestations that are hazardous or dangerous to the self or others, social and antisocial behaviors, and current levels of treatment and medication.

For the purposes of this study, patients evaluated over a one-month period were considered to be representative of the mix of patients to be found in any given facility. Since the instrument from which our own checklist was derived was designed basically to provide a profile of the physical and mental health of a facility's patients, the results reported here are aggregated data and do not yield information on individual patients' conditions.

Data collection

All patients in the seven Massachusetts state mental hospitals were evaluated by data collectors who had received special training from the Director of Research and a team of psychiatric nurses from the Department of Mental Health. Training sessions were devoted to item-by-item explanations of the instrument and methods for its completion. Actual patient assessments were completed by a team consisting of a psychiatric nurse, a psychologist or social worker, and a mental health assistant. Reliability was attained through consensus among raters. In addition, an on-site audit was carried out two weeks after data collection had begun, at which time the psychiatric nurse member of the investigative team met with clinical staff at the hospital unit to review progress and to audit completed patient assessments.

Data analysis

Frequency distributions were completed for each of the key demographic variables. This was followed by an analysis of covariance by sex, while controlling for age, for activities of daily living variables, for aggressive and psychotic behaviors, and for clinical intervention variables.

Demographic, Socioeconomic, and Diagnostic Differences

Demographic differences

The population consisted of 1,042 men and 856 women, and our data confirmed earlier findings in showing a variety of demographic differences by gender. Men in our hospitalized group were very significantly overrepresented in the younger age groups and women were overrepresented in the older age groups (Table 1). The mean age for men was 43 ± 17.8 years, as contrasted with 52 ± 18.5 years for females. Because of this wide age discrepancy and our interest in focusing primarily on illness-related issues, all except demographic data were adjusted for age.

Socioeconomic differences

Table 2 displays data on education, employment, and marriage for male and female patients. Findings related to marriage and educational level were consistent with the generally noted earlier age of onset of schizophrenia among males: 41 percent of the women were or had been married compared with only 20 percent of the men ($p = 0.0001$). Women had also achieved higher educational levels: 41 percent of them were high school graduates compared with 36 percent of the men ($p = 0.017$).

TABLE 1. Age Distribution of State Hospital Inpatients by Sex: 1983

	Men ($n = 1,042$)		Women ($n = 856$)	
Age	Count	%	Count	%
0–21	58	5.6	34	4.0
22–34	364	34.9	157	18.4
35–44	202	19.4	119	13.8
45–64	243	23.3	324	37.8
65+	175	16.8	222	26.0

$\chi^2 = 109, 467$; $df = 4$; $p = 0.0001$

TABLE 2. Education, Employment, and Marital Status of State Hospital Inpatients by Sex: 1983

Socioeconomic Status	Men		Women	
	Count	**%**	**Count**	**%**
Education[a]				
Less than high school	382	45.2	267	38.1
High school	301	35.6	289	41.3
College	162	19.2	144	20.6
$\chi^2 = 8,144$; $df = 2$; $p = 0.017$				
Ever Employed				
Never employed	315	30.2	255	29.8
Employed	727	69.8	601	70.2
χ^2 = not significant				
Ever Married				
Never married	819	79.6	508	59.3
Married	213	20.4	348	40.7
$\chi^2 = 92.21$; $df = 1$; $p = 0.0001$				

[a] Data not available for 197 men and 156 women.

Diagnostic differences

Table 3 presents diagnostic distributions for men and women in the study population and indicates that women had affective illness diagnoses more often than men (16.6 percent as opposed to 8.5 per-

TABLE 3. Diagnosis by Sex in Massachusetts State Hospitals: 1983

Diagnosis[a]	Men		Women	
	Count	**%**	**Count**	**%**
Schizophrenia	703	68.8	527	62.4
Major affective	87	8.5	140	16.6
Other	112	11.0	80	9.5
Retardation	120	11.7	97	11.5
$\chi^2 = 28.412$; $df = 3$; $p = 0.0001$.				

[a] Data not available for 20 men and 12 women.

cent). Men, however, were diagnosed as schizophrenic more often than women (68.8 percent as opposed to 62.4 percent). Mental retardation and a general "other" diagnostic category including personality disorders, neurological disorders, and substance abuse were equally distributed between men and women.

Table 4 provides additional data on age for schizophrenic patients, who constituted more than three-fifths of the study population for both men and women. Fifty-seven percent of the schizophrenic population consisted of men. Moreover, the younger age groupings within that population (under 45 years) also consisted primarily of men. However, among the older age groupings (over 45), women predominated slightly.

By contrast, Table 5 shows that 62 percent of all patients diagnosed with affective disorders were women. The sexes tended to be somewhat equally distributed in the middle and younger age groups. However, women predominated substantially in the age groupings over 45. In the over 65 group women accounted for nearly 80 percent of the population diagnosed with these disorders.

Behavioral and Treatment Differences

While our demographic, socioeconomic, and diagnostic findings support what has previously been reported in the literature, our data on behavioral and treatment differences among male and female state hospital patients indicate some new directions. Table 6 shows a number of statistically significant differences among men and women according to a variety of such behavioral and treatment variables.

Of particular note is the fact that men were more physically threatening with homicidal threats ($p = 0.03$), more sexually threatening ($p = 0.002$), and more sexually assaultive ($p = 0.002$) than women. It should also be noted that these data may actually understate men's tendencies toward frequent physical threats and violence, because Massachusetts has a separate state facility for men who require higher levels of security, but no such facility for women. Accordingly, most chronically mentally ill men considered to be acutely homicidal or otherwise imminently dangerous to others are not represented in the study population.

On the other hand, suicide attempts and threats, sleep disturbances, physical abuse of self, and danger to self (all at $p = 0.001$)

TABLE 4. Schizophrenic Patients Classified by Age and Sex: 1983

Sex	No. (%) of Patients in Age Group					
	Under 22	22–34	35–44	45–64	65+	Total
Male	31 (62.0)	248 (73.2)	135 (64.9)	154 (45.2)	135 (46.2)	703 (57.2)
Female	19 (38.0)	91 (26.8)	73 (35.1)	187 (54.8)	157 (53.8)	527 (42.8)

$\chi^2 = 74.80$; $df = 4$; $p = 0.0001$

TABLE 5. Major Affective Disorder Patients Classified by Age and Sex: 1983

Sex	No. (%) of Patients in Age Group					
	Under 22	22–34	35–44	45–64	65+	Total
Male	6 (54.5)	34 (53.1)	13 (50.0)	25 (30.5)	9 (20.5)	87 (38.3)
Female	5 (45.5)	30 (46.9)	13 (50.0)	57 (69.5)	35 (79.5)	140 (61.7)

$\chi^2 = 16.730$; $df = 4$; $p = 0.0022$

TABLE 6. Analysis of Covariance of Behavioral and Treatment Variables by Sex (Adjusted for Age): 1983

Behavioral or Treatment Variable	Adjusted Mean		F	Significance of F*
	Men	Women		
Typical During Last Three Months				
Suicide attempts	1.13	1.25	17.31	0.0001*
Suicide threats	1.22	1.41	24.43	0.0001*
Homicide attempts	1.13	1.10	1.34	0.24
Homicide threats	1.38	1.30	4.45	0.03*
Dangerous to self	1.76	2.01	18.43	0.0001*
Dangerous to others	1.86	1.81	0.90	0.34
At Least Once During Last Month				
Fire hazard	1.19	1.14	3.75	0.053
Destroy property	1.54	1.61	2.69	0.10
Physically abuse self	1.48	1.71	23.9	0.0001*
Physically abuse others	1.82	1.91	3.23	0.07
Sexually assault others	1.14	1.07	9.42	0.002*
Sexually threaten others	1.23	1.13	8.90	0.002*
Escape	1.47	1.44	0.46	0.49

Behavioral Differences Between Female and Male Patients

	At Least Once a Week			
Severely withdrawn	2.26	2.17	2.51	0.11
Hallucinations	2.22	2.25	0.34	0.55
Temper tantrums	2.18	2.64	68.03	0.0001*
Antisocial disposal of excreta	1.21	1.27	3.53	0.06
Excessive ingestion of foreign substances	1.16	1.17	0.20	0.65
Disrobe/expose self	1.32	1.51	22.15	0.0001*
Sexually disrupt others	1.33	1.31	0.24	0.62
Wander	1.54	1.54	0.01	0.91
	At Least Daily			
Verbally abuse others	2.01	2.31	30.5	0.0001*
Otherwise disrupt others	2.02	2.38	43.7	0.0001*
Problematic sleeping behavior	1.53	1.80	39.72	0.0001*
Hoard	1.29	1.39	6.27	0.01*
	Treatment Variable			
Requires physical restraint	1.50	1.51	0.01	0.90
Requires chemical restraint	1.54	1.70	13.01	0.0003*
Intervention of psychiatrist	2.08	2.27	6.09	0.01*
Intervention of interdisciplinary team	3.83	4.16	10.66	0.001*

*$p \leq 0.05$.

occurred more frequently in women than in men. Women also had significantly more occurrences of temper tantrums, verbal abuse, disrobing, and otherwise disruptive behaviors (all at $p = 0.0001$).

The women in our study also were found to require chemical restraint more often ($p = 0.0003$) and to receive more frequent psychiatric ($p = 0.01$) and interdisciplinary team ($p = 0.0001$) interventions than did the men.

Not shown in Table 6 are those data categories in which no or few significant gender differences were found after adjustment for age. These nonsignificant differences were found in activities of daily living (bathing, dressing, feeding, ambulation, toileting, and so forth) and the ability to adjust to the environment, including handling personal possessions, space, and privileges). Women, however, were generally found to be less cooperative with staff in treatment programs and less able to maintain self-medication programs.

Discussion

The results reported in this study represent a preliminary investigation of gender differences in a large statewide population of hospitalized chronically mentally ill individuals. These data corroborate earlier findings on demographic, socioeconomic, and diagnostic variables.

Beyond this, our results demonstrate that, even though there may not be measurable gender-related differences in daily living skills among chronically mentally ill inpatients in state mental hospitals, this is not necessarily the case for other behavioral expressions of illness or for certain kinds of treatment variables.

We should like to offer some hypotheses to explain the differences we found in gender-related behavioral and treatment variables to set the stage for further research. Toward that end we shall attempt to analyze our findings within the context of the emerging literature on differences in male and female development and psychology.

During the past several years, theories of female development and psychology based on observations of and data about women have been emerging (11–15). These theories are unlike earlier ones in that past developmental theories about women were largely derived from observations of men. Women were seen as exceptions to, or deviant from, "normal" (that is, male) development.

In contrast to the older theories that "posit some form of autonomy or separation as the developmental path" (14), the newer theories focus on "growth within relationship or . . . 'self-in-relation'" among women (14). In short, women increasingly are being seen as developing and existing in their connectedness to others and as defining themselves through their participation in, and striving for, meaningful interactions. This understanding contrasts with the male prototype of development that occurs through increasing emotional and physical independence and self-sufficiency.

It is possible to hypothesize that our findings on female behaviors represent pathological equivalents of seeking for self-definition in relationships, that is, in interactions with others. It is notable that, in a population in which more than 60 percent of the members are chronic schizophrenic patients, the women still appear to be significantly more interactive than the men: They demand more attention and time from those around them. By contrast, the males tend to be more physically threatening and assaultive in their expressions of illness and less verbally interactive. These differences may be interpreted as gender-differentiated expressions of behavior distorted by the disease process.

When interpreted in this way, our findings suggest strongly that sensitivity to such gender differences should inform the planning of services and treatments for chronic mental patients. In general, women might benefit from structured opportunities to interact with staff and patients, to express themselves, and to learn to listen to others; while men might benefit from interventions that are not primarily verbal and that are designed to foster control over physical impulses. Similarly, rehabilitative programs for women might attempt to encourage and validate discussion of self in relation to others, while those for men might focus more on encouraging a sense of independence and autonomy to the highest degree possible.

The planning of physical environments might also reflect gender differences. Spaces that permit and encourage private, quiet conversation might be appropriate for many female patients. It might be well to attempt to separate these spaces from areas provided for physical activities and television watching.

There are even staffing implications that follow from these interpretations of our data. For example, since there is a strong indication that women have significantly more sleep disturbances than men, it may be important not to assume that they will sleep through the night and to provide programs in which staff members are available to talk with them around the clock.

Conclusions

The results of our study of the universe of chronically mentally ill individuals in Massachusetts state mental hospitals strongly emphasize the fact that chronic mental illnesses, while devastating, do not eradicate behavioral differences among individuals in general, or more specifically, between women and men. Whether biologically or culturally derived, gender identification continues to influence role expectations and behaviors. Chronic mental illness tends to be expressed within the context of such differences.

Our data strongly indicate both the need for future research and possible directions that that research might take. Further studies are needed to corroborate our findings, to establish additional gender-related differences in behavior and treatment needs among chronically mentally ill individuals, and to assess the outcomes of therapeutic interventions designed specifically to respond to those differences.

References

1. Bachrach LL: Deinstitutionalization and women. Am Psychol 39:1171–1177, 1984
2. Bachrach LL: Chronic mentally ill women: emergence and legitimation of program issues. Hosp Community Psychiatry 36:1063–1069, 1984
3. Test MA, Berlin SB: Issues of special concern to chronically mentally ill women. Professional Psychology 12:136–145, 1981
4. Forrest AD, Hay AJ: Sex differences and the schizophrenic experience. Acta Psychiatr Scand 47:137–149, 1971
5. Flor-Henry P: Psychosis, neurosis, and epilepsy. Br J Psychiatry 124:144–150, 1974
6. Tudor W, Tudor JF, Grove WR: The effect of sex role differences on the social control of mental illness. J Health Social Behav 18:98–112, 1977
7. Lewine RRJ: Sex differences in schizophrenia: a commentary. Schizophrenia Bull 5:4–7, 1979

8. Lewine RRJ: Sex differences in age of symptom onset and first hospitalization in schizophrenia. Am J Psychiatry 50:316–322, 1980

9. Seeman MV: Interaction of sex, age, and neuroleptic dose. Compr Psychiatry 24:125–128, 1983

10. Seeman MV: Schizophrenic men and women require different treatment programs. Journal of Psychiatric Treatment and Evaluation 5:143–148, 1983

11. Miller JB: Toward A New Psychology of Women. Boston, Beacon Press, 1976

12. Gilligan C: In a Different Voice. Cambridge, Harvard University Press, 1982

13. Kaplan AG: Female or male psychotherapists for women: new formulations. Work in Progress no. 5. Stone Center Working Paper Series. Wellesley, MA, 1984

14. Kaplan AG: "Self-in-relation": implications for depression in women. Work in Progress no. 14. Stone Center Working Paper Series. Wellesley, MA, 1984

15. Stiver IP: The meanings of "dependency" in female-male relationships. Work in Progress no. 11. Stone Center Working Paper Series. Wellesley, MA, 1984

Chapter 4

Women and Work: After Psychiatric Hospitalization

PAULA GOERING, R.N., Ph.D.
JEANETTE COCHRANE, B.A. Hon.
HARRY POTASZNIK, M.A.
DONALD WASYLENKI, M.D., M.Sc.
WILLIAM LANCEE, M.Sc.

Chapter 4

Women and Work: After Psychiatric Hospitalization

That gender role stereotypes permeate all areas of our lives is by this time axiomatic. It is not surprising, then, that the chronically mentally ill women is subject to the same pervasive societal patterns. The authors of this chapter document the paucity of data available about a central area of concern for women—their work. The 260 women followed for six months after discharge from the hospital had unmet needs for employment services to help them find and keep jobs. This may be a critical, generally unaddressed factor in eventual outcome and rehabilitation.

*F*or most of us, work plays a central part in our lives. Our work provides us with meaningful and rewarding activity and contributes significantly to our self-identity and self-esteem. Freud's axiom that the ability to love and to work are the criteria of mental health makes as much sense to us now in the late twentieth century as it did in his time. Given the importance work has in our society in general, it is appropriate to examine what part it plays in the lives of women disabled by psychiatric disorder.

If one turns to the psychiatric research literature to increase understanding of this topic, it is striking how little information is available about the work lives of female psychiatric patients. We became aware of this fact a couple of years ago when we conducted a literature search for studies of employment among women with psychiatric disorders. The search was in response to a consultation request from Employment and Immigration Canada. This federal agency was interested in the possibility of funding employment services targeted for psychiatrically disabled women. It sought our assistance in conducting a needs assessment to determine what types of services might be required by whom.

One of the first steps in a needs assessment is the identification and description of the target population. Our consultee agency made clear that it was interested in "employable" patients who were sufficiently severely ill to be considered disabled. These criteria were broadly operationalized defined as covering hospitalized women with recent histories of employment. But these broad criteria left many questions unanswered. Should the needs assessment be focused on women in particular treatment settings or should it be limited to those with short-term illness histories and less severe (that is, nonpsychotic) diagnoses? Was the posthospital period an appropriate time to offer services? Was there evidence of unmet service needs and, if so, what type of specialized services for women might be required?

Our first response to the agency's request for expert assistance in answering these questions was to conduct a comprehensive review of studies of posthospital outcome and vocational services for psychiatric patients. We found very few studies with specific information about employed women (1, 2), in contrast to numerous studies of male subjects (3–7). The employment experiences of depressed women have received the most attention (8–10), but the majority of these studies are based on outpatient or community samples. There are only a handful of reports that focus on the employment of more severely ill women, and they report on small numbers of subjects (11, 12).

Our second response to the request was to analyze the data from a follow-up study of discharged patients that included extensive information about the employment patterns and problems of 260 women subjects. Before describing the results of that study, we should like to give some consideration to possible reasons for the paucity of investigations of the working lives of women patients.

Bachrach (13) and others (14, 15) have described how sexual role stereotypes that minimize the importance of paid work for women can act as barriers to employment planning by mental health professionals. The same stereotypes may restrict the focus of research. The relative inattention to the work lives of women in comparison to those of men is also present in occupational stress studies of the general population. Even though women make up close to 50 percent of the labor force, we know very little about their work-related problems. For every study in the previous decade concerning women and occupational stress, there have been roughly six concerning men (16). For both psychiatric patients and women in general, the scope of our scientific investigations does not adequately reflect the dramatic change in women's role in the workplace. A preoccupation with comparisons of employed women and housewives suggests that our society is still struggling with the question of whether women "should" work rather than accepting the reality of women working outside the home and attempting to understand its implications.

Another major obstacle to studies of work and psychiatrically disabled women is methodological rather than attitudinal. The definition of women's work role is more complex than that for men. The shifts in our society toward women playing a larger part in the workplace have not been accompanied by a similar shift with regard to men's role in the home. This means that for women, work is not synonymous with employment. Many women work at home in addition to or instead of paid employment. Some researchers include considerations of both domestic and employment work roles for women subjects (11, 17), but there are no standard methods of defining and weighting the multiple role possibilities.

The objective of this study was to provide information that would help to define and describe the target population for a needs assessment of employment services for psychiatrically disabled women. The specific questions addressed were:

1. What proportion of women hospitalized for psychiatric treatment are employed? To what extent do diagnosis, treatment history, or treatment setting define the population?
2. During the posthospital period, are there changes in employment status? What job difficulties and vocational service use occur?
3. Do the employment patterns and problems of women differ from those of men?

Methods

The data were gathered as a part of a larger study of psychiatric aftercare in metropolitan Toronto that has been described in detail in previous reports (18, 19).

49

Procedure

During a six-month period we approached all patients consecutively admitted to 12 psychiatric wards in four different hospitals in metropolitan Toronto: a research institute, a provincial hospital, and two general hospitals. Shortly after their discharge, we interviewed hospital staff and administered an author-constructed scale to inquire about discharge needs and referrals relating to five components of aftercare including vocational/educational. Six months posthospital, we conducted a personal interview, usually in the subject's home. This interview was semistructured and involved inquiries about the use of aftercare services throughout the six-month period, as well as the subjects' social functioning and levels of symptomatology. Instruments included a Social Functioning Schedule (20), the Brief Psychiatric Rating Scale (21), and a Brief Follow-up Rating Scale (22). Only the latter scale was used in a 24-month follow-up interview.

Data analysis

Contingency analysis (chi-square or Fisher's exact test where appropriate) and a significance level of 0.05 were utilized to test differences.

Sample

Subjects in this study represented approximately 14 percent of the total number of patients discharged for the entire system of psychiatric services in metropolitan Toronto. There were 747 subjects in the discharge sample, 505 in the six-month follow-up, and 488 in the two-year follow-up. This report focuses on the 260 women in the six-month follow-up sample. Their demographic and treatment characteristics are summarized in Tables 1 and 2.

The majority of the subjects were between the ages of 25 and 45 with high school educations. Only one-third were married. One-third were immigrants to Canada. Depending upon whether one uses the criterion of diagnosis or treatment history to define the chronically mentally ill, from 27 to 66 percent of the sample might qualify. (A separate analysis of the subgroup of female subjects with

TABLE 1. Demographic Characteristics of Hospitalized Women (*n* = 260)

Characteristic	No.	(%)
Age (yr)		
≤25	52	(20)
26–45	129	(50)
≥46	79	(30)
Education		
University	44	(17)
High school	148	(57)
Grade school	68	(26)
Marital Status		
Single	110	(42)
Married	81	(31)
Separated/divorced	53	(20)
Widowed	16	(6)
Birthplace		
Canada	178	(69)
Other	82	(32)

neurotic diagnoses [23] suggests that many of them also have long-term and severe impairments in social functioning.)

TABLE 2. Treatment Characteristics of Hospitalized Women (*n* = 260)

Characteristic	No.	(%)
Admitting Diagnosis		
Schizophrenia	66	(25)
Other psychosis	66	(25)
Neurosis	87	(34)
Personality disorder and alcoholism	41	(16)
No. of Previous Admissions		
None	64	(25)
1–5	127	(49)
More than 5	69	(27)
Hospital		
Research institute	44	(17)
Provincial hospital	97	(37)
Downtown general hospital	44	(17)
Suburban general hospital	75	(29)
Type of Admission		
Informal	214	(82)
Involuntary	46	(18)

Results

Relationship of Hospitalization and
Type of Treatment to Employment Status

Thirty-five percent of the 260 women subjects in the sample were employed in full- or part-time work before hospital admission. Another 26 percent had been employed within the previous two years. Six months later, 40 percent (105 women) were employed; 24 months later 28 percent were employed.

The 105 women employed at the six-month follow-up were in a variety of occupations, with the majority in clerical or sales positions and 29 percent in unskilled jobs. Only 17 percent were doing part-time work. Thirty-six percent of the employed women were living with a spouse and/or children and had major household responsibilities in addition to their paid employment.

Treatment setting did not predict posthospital employment, but, as is shown in Table 3, there were some diagnostic and treatment characteristics that differentiated the employed from the unemployed. Subjects with a neurotic diagnosis and those with fewer than five previous admissions were more likely to be employed. Still, it should be noted that 32 to 38 percent of those with more severe diagnoses and 31 percent of those with numerous prior admissions were in the employed group. Diagnosis was generally unre-

TABLE 3. Treatment Characteristics That Differentiate Employed and Unemployed Women Six Months Posthospital ($n = 260$)

Characteristic	No.	Employment Rate (%)
Diagnosis		
Schizophrenia	66	34
Other psychosis	66	38
Neurosis	87	52**
Personality disorder and alcoholism	41	32
No. of Previous Admissions		
None	64	48
1–5	127	42
More than 5	69	31*

*$p \geq 0.05$ by Fisher's exact test; **$p \geq 0.01$ by Fisher's exact test.

lated to type of employment, except that a higher proportion (37 percent) of schizophrenic subjects were in unskilled jobs.

Change in Employment Status, Job Difficulties, and Vocational Service Use

There was no change in the preadmission and six-month follow-up employment status of 73 percent of the sample population. Twelve percent of the women lost employment, and 15 percent gained employment. A chart review was completed of those two change subgroups. Only a few of the women who gained employment did so with the assistance of service agencies. Most had unstable work histories and had moved in and out of employment frequently. A similar pattern of employment instability was evident for some of those who had lost jobs, but others in this group reported being fired because of their illness and hospitalization(s). There was a relationship between rehospitalization and employment status. Thirty percent of the rehospitalized women ($n = 94$) were employed, whereas 48 percent of those not rehospitalized were employed.

Table 4 shows how employed women ranked reported areas of difficulty with social functioning. There are two subscales of the Social Functioning Schedule concerned with work. The work behavior subscale asks about difficulties in completing tasks and doing the

TABLE 4. Areas of Difficulty with Social Functioning Reported by Employed Women ($n = 105$)

Area	% Reporting Difficulty
Social relationships	64
Marital relationships[a]	50
Work (stress)	48
Leisure (behavior)	48
Finances (stress)	48
Leisure (stress)	46
Household chores (behavior)	29
Finances (behavior)	28
Household chores (stress)	24
Work (behavior)	22

[a] $n = 30$.

53

job well. Twenty-two percent of the employed women reported moderate or major difficulties with work behavior. The work stress subscale asks about difficulties in getting along with people at work, feeling worried and upset by things that happen at work, or feeling bored or dissatisfied. Almost one-half of the employed subjects reported moderate or major difficulties in this area.

Diagnosis, number of previous admissions, and type of job were unrelated to difficulties at work. There was, however, an association between severity of symptoms and difficulties with both work behavior and work stress. Employed subjects with low symptom levels six months posthospital ($n = 45$) were much less likely to be having difficulty with work behavior (7 percent) or work stress (27 percent).

At discharge, hospital staff identified needs for vocational/educational services for 36 percent of the 260 women subjects. The identified need were for vocational assessment, placement, and training services. Only one-half of those with identified needs received referrals. The most common reasons given for not making a referral were that the patient was not motivated, was not ready, or had indicated she would do it on her own. Six months later, 23 percent of women subjects had made contact with a vocational/educational service some time during the six-month period.

Employment Patterns and Problems of Women and Men

The demographic and treatment characteristics of the male and female subjects in this sample differ only with regard to diagnosis and treatment setting. Women were more likely to have a diagnosis of neurosis and to be hospitalized in a general hospital.

There were no differences across or within diagnostic categories in the rates of employment. However, for all diagnoses, men were more likely to be employed in skilled or semiskilled occupations, whereas women were more likely to be in clerical or sales positions. There were no sex differences in patterns of service use, changes in employment status, or reported difficulties, except that within the diagnostic category of "other psychosis" (composed primarily of psychotic depressions) women reported less difficulty with work behavior and stress than did men.

Even though there were no sex differences in rates of employment in the study sample, if one compares the employment rates

Women and Work: After Psychiatric Hospitalization

TABLE 5. Sex Differences In Employment Rates for Psychiatric Sample and General Population

Population	% Employed (Full or Part Time)	
	Men	Women
Metropolitan Toronto general population ($n = 1,724,925$)[a]	77.5	57.5
Psychiatric sample ($n = 505$)	31.7	40.4

[a]*Statistics Canada*, 1981

with those in the general population (Table 5), the discrepancy is considerably greater for the male subjects.

Another difference between men and women subjects with regard to vocational outcome is that housewives are a distinct subgroup that may have unique needs for vocational/educational services. Table 6 illustrates that the housewives are less well educated than either employed women or those who are unemployed and without household responsibilities. They are not as severely ill or as impaired as the unemployed and are having less difficulty with social relationships than the employed.

TABLE 6. Selected Predictors and Correlates[a] of Work Outcome for Discharged Women

Predictor or Correlate	% of Women:			
	Employed ($n = 105$)	Housewives ($n = 59$)	Not Working ($n = 96$)	Total ($n = 260$)
Grade school education	17	47	23	26
Neurotic diagnosis	52	31	17	34
No previous admissions	49	32	19	25
High symptoms	21	23	41	29
Readmitted	27	37	49	37
Difficulties with social relationships	64	43	74	63

[a] χ^2 analysis, $p < 0.05$.

Discussion

Employment was clearly a pertinent issue for a considerable number of the women hospitalized for psychiatric treatment. Since the majority were employed or had recent work histories, a needs assessment for employment services that focused upon a hospitalized population seemed feasible and warranted.

The findings of this study do not support the strategy of focusing a needs assessment on particular treatment settings or limiting interest to those women with short-term histories and less severe diagnoses. Even though there was a relationship between diagnosis and treatment history and the likelihood of employment, the relationship was not strong enough to exclude psychotic individuals or those with more than five admissions from consideration. The finding that schizophrenic subjects were more likely to be employed in unskilled occupations suggests that diagnosis may have more implications for the quality and type of work performance than it does for employment per se (4, 24).

The results of this study indicate that there were unmet needs for employment services during the period after discharge. The number of women utilizing services was considerably fewer than the number assessed by the hospital staff to be in need. The needs identified at discharge were primarily for those who were unemployed and seeking employment. If one assumes that subjects who lost employment after discharge and those who experienced difficulties at work were also in need of employment services, the amount of unmet need was even greater.

Interventions aimed at helping to keep jobs may be as important as those aimed at finding employment. The nature of the difficulties reported by the employed women suggests that social skills or assertiveness training and stress management techniques focused on occupational stressors may be particularly valuable. Our findings also point to the importance of illness management when considering employment. Rehospitalization and high levels of symptoms had negative associations with vocational outcome.

Sex differences in vocational outcome were examined to assess whether specialized employment services may be needed for women. For the most part, there were no differences in vocational outcome between the male and female subjects.

The absence of difference in employment rates and the delineation of housewives as a separate outcome group are the findings with the greatest implications for service planning. Before we discuss these issues, we shall give brief consideration to the sex differences we did find in occupation and in impairment within one diagnostic group.

Others have reported, as we do, that women patients are more likely to be in white-collar and men in blue-collar jobs (17, 25). As Freeman and Simmons (25) point out, this distribution reflects sex differences in the occupations of the lower socioeconomic class of the general population. Our findings about impairment are similar to those of a study of psychiatric outpatients. Weissman and co-workers (26) found no sex differences in employment rates or impairment except that depressed women were less impaired than depressed men. That is consistent with the results of this study, since the diagnostic category "other psychosis" is composed primarily of those with affective disorders. Working outside of the home may provide unique positive benefits—for example, escape, protection, or distraction—for depressed women (8).

Studies of vocational outcome that report on sex differences generally find women as likely to be employed as men (27, 28). It is only when one compares the employment rates of the psychiatric sample to those of the general population, where men predominate, that sex differences appear. In this study, the larger discrepancy for men between the employment rates of the psychiatric sample and those of the general population do not appear to be explained by men's having an earlier age of onset and poorer premorbid functioning (29). There were no sex differences in age or education across or within diagnostic categories.

It is possible that stigma creates a greater obstacle to obtaining employment for male psychiatric patients than it does for female patients. A study of worker acceptance of former mental patients found that men were treated more poorly than women even when they had identical psychiatric histories (30). Similar findings of greater rejection of men are reported in studies of schizophrenia, depression, and social attraction (31, 32). One explanation is that women patients are seen as less aggressive and less potentially dangerous. The different responses may also reflect societal attitudes that pathological emotional behavior is more acceptable in women than men (33). Whatever the explanation, it appears that female patients seeking employment may have an advantage over men in this regard.

Just as men may require specialized assistance in dealing with stigma, women may require specialized support services in order both to work and to carry out their household responsibilities. Housewives in this study are less impaired than the unemployed and probably have a greater potential for vocational success, if the necessary transportation, childcare, and homemaking services were available. Educational upgrading and job training are other services that are probably required (12).

Note should be taken of the group of women who were employed and held major household responsibilities. A comparison of their characteristics, service use, and functioning with those of the other employed subjects revealed no significant differences. The ability to continue to fulfill their multiple obligations after an acute episode of illness and hospitalization indicates considerable strength and resiliency. The capacity to be ill and to continue to function is a common female attribute. It is a capacity that deserves recognition and further investigation.

Summary

Data from a follow-up study that included 260 women hospitalized for psychiatric disorder have been analyzed to identify and describe a target population for a needs assessment of employment services. We found that employment was a pertinent issue for large numbers of this population, including those with severe diagnoses and chronic treatment histories. Unmet needs for service use in the posthospital period were evident. The implications for service planning of differences in the employment patterns and problems of men and women have been discussed.

The results of this study provide quantitative information that only begins to describe the employment status of psychiatrically disabled women. Although planning services on the basis of the results of a few studies is better than planning in a vacuum, our knowledge about this subject is far from adequate. Employment is an important issue for women as well as men. More attention needs to be paid to understanding the part it plays in the lives of women with psychiatric disorders.

References

1. Brodsky C: The social recovery of mentally ill housewives. Family Process 7:170–183, 1968
2. Douzinas N, Carpenter M: Predicting the community performance of vocational rehabilitation clients. Hosp Community Psychiatry 32:409–413, 1981
3. Bean LL: Mental illness and occupational adjustment: a 10 year follow-up study. Soc Sci Med 2:435–446, 1968
4. Cole NJ, Shupe DR: A four-year follow-up of former psychiatric patients in industry. Arch Gen Psychiatry 22:222–229, 1970
5. Huffine CL, Clausen JA: Madness and work: short- and long-term effects of mental illness on occupational careers. Social Forces 57:1049–1062, 1979
6. Lipton H, Kaden SE: Predicting the posthospital work adjustment of married, male schizophrenics. Journal of Consulting Psychology 29:93, 1965
7. Lorei TW, Gurel L: Demographic characteristics as predictors of post-hospital employment and readmission. J Consult Clin Psychol 40:426–430, 1973
8. Mostow E, Newberry P: Work role and depression in women: a comparison of workers and housewives in treatment. Am J Orthopsychiatry 45:538–548, 1975
9. Weissman MM, Paybel S: The Depressed Woman: A Study of Social Relationships. Chicago, University of Chicago Press, 1974
10. Wetzel JW, Richmond FC: A person-environment study of depression. Social Service Review 54:363–375, 1980
11. Holstein A: Women, work and mental health: the interaction between work relationships and psychiatric illness. Master's Thesis. New Haven, CT, Yale University School of Nursing, 1984
12. Test MA, Berlin S: Issues of special concern to chronically mentally ill women. Professional Psychology 12:136–145, 1981
13. Bachrach LL: Chronic mentally ill women: emergence and legitimation of program issues. Hosp Community Psychiatry 36:1063–1069, 1985
14. Carmen EH, Russo NF, Miller JBK: Inequality and women's mental health: an overview. Am J Psychiatry 138:1319–1330, 1981

15. Zeldow PB: Sex differences in psychiatric evaluation and treatment. Arch Gen Psychiatry 35:89–93, 1978
16. Haw MA: Women, work and stress: a review and agenda for the future. J Health Soc Behav 23:132–144, 1982
17. Kinard EM, Klerman LV: Changes in life style following mental hospitalization. J Nerv Ment Dis 168:666–672, 1981
18. Goering P, Wasylenki D, Lancee W, et al: From hospital to community six-month and two-year outcomes for 505 patients. J Nerv Ment Dis 172:667–673, 1984
19. Wasylenki D, Goering P, Lancee W, et al: Psychiatric aftercare in a metropolitan setting. Can J Psychiatry 30:329–336, 1985
20. Remington M, Tyrer P: The social functioning schedule: a brief semi-structured interview. Social Psychiatry 14:151–157, 1979
21. Overall JE, Gorham DR: The brief psychiatric rating scale. Psychol Rep 10:799–812, 1962
22. Soskis DA: A brief follow-up rating scale. Compr Psychiatry 11:445–449, 1970
23. Goering P, Wasylenki D, Lancee W, et al: Social support and post hospital outcome for depressed women. Can J Psychiatry 28:612–618, 1983
24. Wansbrough N, Cooper P: Open Employment After Mental Illness. London, Tavistock Publications, 1980
25. Freeman HE, Simmons OG: The Mental Patient Comes Home. New York, John Wiley, 1963
26. Weissman MM, Prusoff BA, Thompson WD, et al: Social adjustment by self-report in a community sample and in psychiatric outpatients. J Nerv Ment Dis 166:317–326, 1978
27. Buell GJ, Anthony WA: Demographic characteristics as predictors of recidivism and post-hospital employment. Journal of Counseling Psychology 20:361–365, 1973
28. Gift TE, Harder DW, Ritzler BA, et al: Sex and race of patients admitted for their first psychiatric hospitalization: correlates and prognostic power. Am J Psychiatry 142:1447–1449, 1985
29. Seeman MV: Gender differences in schizophrenia. Can J Psychiatry 27:107–112, 1982
30. Farina A, Murray PJ, Groh T: Sex and worker acceptance of a former mental patient. J Consult Clin Psychol 46:887–891, 1978
31. Boswell PC, Murray EJ: Depression, schizophrenia and social attraction. J Consult Clin Psychol 49:641–647, 1981

32. Hammen CL, Peters SD: Differential responses to male and female depressive reactions. J Consult Clin Psychol 45:994–1001, 1977
33. Broverman IK, Broverman DM, Clarkson FE, et al: Sex-role stereotypes and clinical judgement of mental health. J Consult Clin Psychol 34:1–7, 1970

Chapter 5

Being Mentally Ill in America: One Female's Experience

DIAN COX LEIGHTON, B.S.

Being Mentally Ill in America: One Female's Experience

This personal account from a former patient emphasizes for those in the field the struggle of patients, their families, and their communities. It is a perspective that must remain in the foreground of our thinking and planning.

Introduction

I was always dependent. Those in the mental health field would probably describe mine as a dependent personality. It is only fair to admit my dependency or past dependency up front, before I discuss how it was played upon and preyed upon in both the private and public mental health systems.

My dependency had already gotten me into a lot of trouble in my life and had been a major factor in causing my, to put it euphemistically, nervous breakdown. It also became a primary symptom of my illness. Ironically, the dependency that led me into an unhealthy situation and eventually into the world of mental illness was used by mental health professionals, whether consciously or unconsciously, to keep me ill. Dependency never had a minor role in my life.

In terms of my mental illness, my dependency was the key that unlocked doors I never wanted opened, never knew existed.

I had a genetic, environmental, and what I choose to call a societal predisposition to mental illness. I had a full-blown pyschotic break with reality in the mid-1970s. In retrospect, I'd be worried if I hadn't broken. I would have had to have been an extremely insensitive person not to have been profoundly marked by what happened to me. Sometimes it almost makes sense to lose your mind. The trigger that broke me was not a quick one. It was a very unfortunate,

© 1986 Dian Cox Leighton.

highly unusual, and long-term episode in my life. In shortened version, I'll just say that someone saw in me a vulnerability, an insecurity, and an extreme dependency. Over time, he taught me to care for him deeply, trust him completely, to the exclusion of all others, even family and friends. As is typical, I didn't recognize at the time that I was being brainwashed. So eventually, as things got worse, I lost my sense of self, my very soul, you might say, and later my mind.

I got out of the situation alive and more or less intact, but, soon after, started coming apart. I broke in a very bad way. Over the five years of my illness in its most nonfunctional state, I saw close to a dozen doctors, took over 20 types of medications, had three hospitalizations and one serious suicide attempt.

During those years and since, I have been given many labels—phobic, paranoid, paranoid schizophrenic, obsessive-compulsive with episodes of psychosis, and manic-depressive. Often it seems the doctor's diagnosis was too readily reached. And the words they used to describe me frightened me, especially that "cancer of the mind" word "schizophrenic." Being called "chronic," as I was, was killing, too. It made me feel so helpless and hopeless. It made me want to give up. That's why as a mental health consumer advocate, I try to help change the terminology from "chronic" to "long-term." It's interesting to note that after I made what they then described as "a miraculous recovery" from the more severe aspects of my illness, these same doctors said I had not been schizophrenic after all. Yet I had been labeled that way—chronically so—and given up on. It makes me wonder about all the others labeled like me.

There's much talk about gaps in the mental health system. I believe there's a serious gap in the attitude of many mental health professionals. Generally speaking, they don't hold out enough hope to any of us considered long-term ill, whether we're male or female.

Doctors

I remember well my first psychiatrist, whom I saw early in my illness and with whom I remained in treatment too long (and who let me). He doubted what I had told him had happened to me because it sounded too bizarre. As he peered over his glasses at me, I'm sure he wrote down "paranoid delusion." Not being believed by the person I was daring to trust to tell this to was devastating. Psychiatrists do hear a lot of wild stories, but they, above all people, should be able to decipher between reality and unreality. After all, isn't that what they're supposed to be helping us, their parents, do when our minds have intermingled the two states?

Still, doctors are human. Perhaps I should be more understanding. The situation I described was hard to believe. The doctor I found later who did help me so much even asked my mother privately if I had not imagined the story I had told her.

Even so, not being believed hurt. It might have happened to me even if I had been male. But I doubt I would have been treated some of the other ways I was as a female. For example, I usually wasn't listened to. I suppose I was considered a hysterical female who needed tranquilizers. And they gave me many. Then when I had grand mal seizures from overmedication, I was written up as an epileptic—to ward off a lawsuit, I guess. Yet I remember crying and begging my first psychiatrist to believe me, to let me talk to him. Instead, pills and "pablum" were pushed across the desk to me. Often that happened with other doctors, too. I was given new and different medications and the same old "pablum" was spooned my way, as if I were a child, not a grown woman with a serious problem.

This condescending attitude was one I encountered regularly with psychiatrists I saw. True, I was hysterical. But my hysteria was too easily accepted, almost expected. I didn't seem to be someone the doctors wanted to communicate with. Instead of being talked to, at times I was actually patted on the head like a pet, not a person. Would they have done that to a male? I doubt it. I'm sure my small stature enlarged their feelings about me. I don't believe I was viewed as strong enough to fight my illness, to get well. In fact, my parents were told to put me away in a state institution—that "people with her thought disorder do not usually recover." Most of the doctors I saw were not ones to tackle my illness head-on or to suggest that I should. They fostered my dependency and I became sicker.

Hospitals

I can't say things were any better for me in the hospital. They weren't. In fact, they were usually worse. And I got worse there. I never actually attempted suicide until after hospitalization. My illness, which was largely one of fear and dependency, increased in the hospital whether I was in a nice, private one or a state institution.

The mothering attempts made by the nurses in the private hospital to get me up and dressed felt condescending and hollow. The only therapy once you were up and dressed was to walk up and down the shiny corridors or sit in the TV room. And there were times in the private hospital when a doctor paid to visit me every day (an advantage to being hospitalized privately) didn't come into my room to see me, although I knew he was on the floor seeing other patients. I was a patient with an aggravating illness—I asked a lot of obsessive-compulsive questions. But I did not need to be dismissed and discounted in such a blunt, hurtful way by the person I thought was supposed to be helping me.

My first stay in a private hospital I had my meals brought to me on a tray and even my medicine. By the time of my second stay, I had progressed and got up and got my own medication. Nothing, however, was taught to me about self-reliance or self-responsibility. No one, from the psychiatrists to the nurses to the aides, indicated that I might have a part in my own illness and wellness.

It was the same in the state institution, only the surroundings were more frightening, which increased my fear and dependency. The main requirement there was to get up and out of bed by 5 a.m. and sit in the day room all day and night until bedtime. There was nothing to do but watch limited staff try to handle the other mental patients. Most of us, though, were so drugged in our chemical straitjackets, we could not do much. I was finally sent to some so-called classes that even in my sick state I found insulting. We were given clay to play with.

While I was in the state institution, a certain nurse was assigned to my case. He clearly didn't like me. Recognizing this dislike, I didn't like him. I felt somehow deep down he was antagonistic toward me. He tried to break my friendship with another woman on the ward. He made fun of me numerous times, referring to me as a baby because I cried. If that technique was to teach self-responsibility, I'm afraid it didn't work. I didn't feel he was very responsible in his treatment of me.

Then one night he did something to me he could only do to a female. He gave me a birth control pill along with my usual medications. I told him I no longer took birth control pills. He answered that it was written up in my charts as one of my medications and that I had to take it until a psychiatrist said I didn't have to. I might add that previous nights while I was there he hadn't given me birth control pills. Why the sudden adherence to the rules? I was afraid to take the pill out of sequence. My illness being one of confusion and fear compounded the problem. I thought taking it out of sequence would harm me in some way. I told him so. He laughed. I told him there was no reason for me to take birth control pills, implying that I didn't have sex. Indeed, I was so afraid of people and men, in particular, that I wouldn't have let anyone touch my arm, much less have sex with me. He didn't seem to care. I cried and begged him not to make me take the pill. Not only did he not seem to care how I felt, he seemed to be enjoying his power over me. State institutions are one of the few places that such power plays can happen. He watched while I tearfully took the pill. I imagined in my sick state that it would kill me. The next day I did arrange with the psychiatrist not to take them.

There seemed to be a prevailing attitude that all females on the ward were promiscuous. That couldn't have been more wrong about me, as I was very frightened of men. Later, after recovery, while working in the mental health field, I found myself relaying the birth control incident to a Volunteer Services Coordinator at the same state hospital. Her reply surprised me, although it shouldn't have. She said, "Why, you were probably promiscuous." Although sex was offered by a male patient for a quarter in the laundry room to any female on the ward, I gave him all my quarters just to be left alone.

While I was on the same ward, a psychiatrist assigned to other patients, not me, began flirting with me. He'd say such things as "Hi, cutie, what are you doing here? You must be one of the workers. You couldn't be a patient." A form of flattery in a state mental institution. His flirting went on day after day. Surely, he wouldn't have been making such comments to a male. He was very familiar with me. I didn't know how to react. If I discouraged him, I was afraid I might make him mad and suffer the consequences. I was afraid he would have me put in lockup or keep me from ever getting out of the hospital. So I would slightly smile at him but I was also afraid to encourage him, knowing I couldn't handle those consequences either and not wanting to. The day came when I was going home—finally. I was so relieved to be getting out and going back to my family. I was at my locker packing up my things when this same psychiatrist came up behind me. He grabbed me by the shoulders, turned me around, said something about my going, and kissed me on the lips. I was too sick still then to be shocked at his lack of professionalism. What struck me was how scared I was that a man had touched me, had kissed me. I had such a fear of this very thing. Sometimes my fear sent me into hysterics. It occurred to me in my disturbed way of thinking that I might die because a man had kissed me. Yet I tried to stand perfectly still and not utter a sound of fear, for this was a doctor. I didn't want to react in any way that might change the minds of the people in charge and have them keep me in the hospital. I didn't tell anyone there what had happened. I just wanted to get away from that man and that place. I wanted to go home.

Today, looking back on his more-than-unprofessional behavior of taking liberties with a mental patient, I'm glad they released me saying I could not adjust to hospital atmosphere. That state institution in Texas in 1977 was not a place a person with any mental health left would want to adjust to.

Two beautiful things did happen to me while I was a patient in the day hospital after release. My mental health worker saw me standing in the hall crying and feeling sorry for myself, which I was so good at doing. She came up to me and said, "What's the matter, Dian? What are you crying for?" I said, "Because I'm mentally ill. Why me, why do I have to be mentally ill?" She just shrugged her shoulders and, walking away, said flippantly to me, "Why am I black?" For the first time in a long time, I stopped and thought about someone else. There was another incident where a social worker teaching a mental health class to us said, "It's not your fault if you're mentally ill, but it is your responsibility to do everything in your power to get well." I was stunned. No one had ever said those words before he had. It both frightened and excited me. I thought there might be a chance after all.

Turning Points

I didn't forget the words I had learned in the day hospital about self-responsibility. And although I saw a number of psychiatrists who didn't encourage me, once I did see a young psychiatrist interning at a public mental health clinic who tried to instill in me a little hope. He dared to suggest that I might be able to turn things around in three years, implying that I might be all right and able to go on with my life. My mother and I couldn't believe it, for we had been told so again. He was unjaded. He was a hopeful doctor. But I didn't get to see him again. He was transferred and I thought that was the end of such encouragement for me.

Not being sophisticated in the mental health system before my years of experience with that system, I had gone to psychiatrists to be "fixed" as one would go to a general practitioner for an antibiotic for an infection. The doctors I saw never told me I had to fix myself and that, at best, they were to serve as good guides. Even when one psychiatrist saw me regressing terribly under his care, he did not refer me to someone else who might be able to better help me. One psychiatrist, however, did send me to a psychologist to supplement his treatment of me. That's how I came to know the doctor who helped me the most.

She was more human than any of the other doctors I had seen and treated me more humanely. There was a rapport and an equality between us—not just because we were the same sex. With the other doctors I had seen, I felt inferior in their presence. Of course, my ego was badly damaged by the illness. But their superior attitudes hurt me even more. This psychologist treated me like one human being helping another. For the first time, strength in me was recognized and fostered. Early in her treatment of me, she let me know I had a responsibility over my own illness and wellness. She insisted that I try, something never suggested previously. Her expectations of me and the hard work she demanded on my part are major reasons I recovered.

I remember the first time I went to see her. I was with my mother because I was afraid to go anywhere without her. The psychologist asked me a lot of questions and really listened to my answers. She was the first mental health professional I had seen who seemed sincerely interested in me as a person, not just another "case." Since I had seen many of the doctors in town, the prognosis wasn't good, and had she seen my records, she may not have held out a great deal of hope. But she gave me a chance, a real chance. At that first meeting, she said she'd work with me for six months. At the end of that time, if we weren't making progress, she wouldn't waste her time or my money. No one had ever cared enough to give me a deadline before. No one had ever been that professional. Amazingly, at the end of six months, I was making a tiny bit of progress.

Therapy with her was real. It was work. Hard work. There is

much discouraging, hopeless news. We were eager for me to see him nothing easy about being mentally ill. There is nothing easy about getting well. But, for some of us, sometimes, with the right kind of guidance, it can happen.

Due to the excellent advice of the psychiatrist I was seeing along with her, I was living away from my family back on my own in an apartment. There was no group home in Austin, Texas, then or any other kind of living arrangement for mental health clients. So I had to struggle without a structure I badly needed.

The psychologist gave me assignments and that helped. One assignment was to walk to her office from my nearby apartment. I usually arrived in a state of panic, so afraid of the very air was I and filled with imaginary, fearful happenings along the way. Yet she kept insisting that I walk. She didn't feed me "pablum," coddle me, or suggest I give up. In other ways, too, she kept pushing me and, more importantly, encouraging me to push myself. When I tried to draw her into my dependency game of answering my questions for reassurance, she answered once, then said, "I'm not Mama and I won't play that game with you." Somehow with her it didn't make me angry. Nor did she listen to my foolish delusions for long—just long enough to let me know she'd heard and then dismiss them. For the first time, I began to let go of some of my obsessions.

With her, I wanted to get well. For I began to believe it could actually happen. She had instilled in me hope. Fighting my own mind—my illness—became a great adventure, a contest with myself. With her, I became less dependent and more determined. I also developed what she called ego strength—a healthy anger at my illness and the mental health system that had failed me.

While mutual support groups are not necessarily a part of the formal mental health system, there is no way I could have made it back to this reality and to an independent existence without them. Neither my last psychiatrist nor psychologist was threatened by them. They saw them as a supplement to their treatment. And my psychiatrist, impressed with the progress I was making with the mutual support group, started a mutual support group in his office, acting only as a resource person. I was then fortunate enough to have two good support groups and two good doctors.

Conclusion

I've been working the past six years in a Texas mental health organization outside the system. I develop, coordinate, and maintain statewide mutual support groups for persons who have or who have had mental or emotional problems, with separate groups for family members and friends of such persons. I promote the project through my personal story. I travel a lot and work long hours. It's a stressful job, but exciting. And I love it. I stay on minimal medication and may have to all my life. I still have a strong dependent streak that I have to constantly guard against. And I don't hesitate to go back and see my psychiatrist or psychologist, if I need to.

In the meantime, I get much support from my understanding husband, mother, and friends. In addition, the words my late grandmother said to me in my years of most despair echo in my memory and help keep me going—"I'm betting on you."

I'm one of the fortunate ones. I learned the hard way that sometimes what happens in the mental health system is not always good for your health. But sometimes it is. And, for me, that's made all the difference.

Chapter 6

Chronic Mentally Ill Women: Emergence and Legitimation of Program Issues

LEONA L. BACHRACH, Ph.D.

Chapter 6

Chronic Mentally Ill Women: Emergence and Legitimation of Program Issues

Program development for chronic mentally ill women is emerging in a climate where more general concerns relating to women's health and mental health are increasingly being examined. Although in the past the special needs of chronic mentally ill women have received scant attention in the professional literature, there is evidence today of a growing commitment to serving this population. The author traces the emergence and legitimation of three specific issues—homelessness, skills training, and family planning—that reflect the complexity of program development for this population. As specific issues in service delivery to chronic mentally ill women come to the fore and move toward relevant solutions, we may anticipate a sharpening of planning concepts. Both male and female chronic mental patients stand to benefit from these developments.

Wilhelmina Franklin was 86 years old, frail, confused, and confined to a wheelchair. Her story has been reported in the *Washington Post* (1, 2). Ms. Franklin froze to death on the grounds of the nursing facility that was her home. Staff members reported not finding her in her room at the nine and ten o'clock bed checks but did not search for her until 11 o'clock. When they found her, she was dead. She was wearing only light clothing, and her wheelchair was tipped over next to her. About 40 years ago Ms. Franklin was admitted to a public mental institution, and about 16 years ago she was

Reprinted with permission from Bachrach LL: Chronically mentally ill women: emergence and legitimation of program issues. Hosp Community Psychiatry 36:1063-1069, 1985.

transferred to the nursing facility where she died. The newspaper report has indicated that Ms. Franklin's death will be studied with extra care because the nursing facility is an integral element in a massive court-ordered deinstitutionalization plan.

Nancy Hopper, aged 27, had a different kind of death. Her story has been reported in the *Boston Globe* (3). Ms. Hopper bled to death from a ruptured ectopic pregnancy over a two-day period during which she was in a seclusion room in a community mental health center. She was what is commonly referred to as a revolving-door patient and was known to a variety of mental health and human service agencies. She was also episodically homeless. She had apparently sought help for abdominal pain at a general hospital emergency room and was referred to the mental health center, where she died.

Judy (no known last name) is a 41-year-old homeless woman who lives on the streets of New York City. Her story has been reported in the *New York Times* (4). She carries a diagnosis of paranoid schizophrenia given her in several court hearings, but she has never actually been hospitalized because she refuses to be committed voluntarily. In the meantime Judy is a vulnerable target who, according to the *Times* article, hallucinates regularly and "scream[s] obscenities into the night." Concerned neighbors want to help and protect Judy but are powerless to do so in the face of her refusal to be hospitalized. One neighbor has said, "Nothing is going to happen until the day someone hurts her."

Ms. A's story has a happier ending but is nonetheless marked by drama and ethical dilemma. The case of Ms. A, a 24-year-old diabetic woman with a history of psychiatric hospitalization for psychotic depression, has been described in the *American Journal of Psychiatry* (5). In her 28th week of pregnancy Ms. A was admitted to the obstetrics and gynecology service of a large urban medical center. During her stay she became increasingly depressed, suicidal, and anorectic, and she required constant attendance. The risk to the fetus from Ms. A's hypoglycemia, and the risk of her suicide, prompted the obstetrical staff, in consultation with psychiatric personnel, to consider treatment with low-voltage ECT—a course that was eventually adopted with considerable reluctance because of uncertainty about its outcome.

The ECT was administered by the hospital's psychiatric consultation staff in the obstetrical unit and in the presence of an obstetrician. After eight sessions Ms. A experienced complete remission of her depressive symptoms but remained hospitalized because of her high-risk pregnancy. She subsequently delivered a normal baby who ten months after birth was judged developmentally normal.

Marcia Lovejoy (6), diagnosed with chronic schizophrenia and now recovered, has related her own story with eloquence and grace in *Hospital and Community Psychiatry*. She has called it a "personal odyssey." To Ms. Lovejoy the treatment system is "woefully inadequate and does not begin to address the need for hopeful and happy lives for those it purports to treat." Today Ms. Lovejoy is executive director of Project Overcome in Minneapolis, a consultation agency and speakers' bureau founded and staffed by former mental patients. She regards her encouragement by a particular psychiatrist who "had hope for me" as a turning point after many years of illness. That psychiatrist, she has written, "believed in me when I did not believe in myself and used multiple approaches in addressing my problems. He sought the answers *with* me rather than *for* me."

The stories of Wilhelmina Franklin, Nancy Hopper, Judy, Ms. A, and Marcia Lovejoy are vignettes in a growing collection of evidence that program development for chronic mentally ill women should be pursued as a separate area of concern. In this article I shall use a conceptual framework proposed by Blumer (7) to examine the evolution of this focal point in service planning.

According to Blumer, the first stage in the career of a social problem is emergence of the issue as a focus of attention. Second, the issue acquires social legitimacy and a "degree of respectability which entitles it to consideration in the recognized arenas of public discussion." Third, there is a mobilization of forces to attack the problem, which is followed, fourth, by the formulation of a plan of action. The final step involves implementing the proposed plan of action.

Emergence of the Problem

Blumer (7) viewed social problems as not resulting simply from "the intrinsic malfunctioning of society" but rather as evolving from "a process of definition in which a given condition is picked out and identified" as problematical. So it is with program development for chronic mentally ill women. A heightened awareness of—and responsiveness to—women's gender-specific treatment needs requires more than a knowledge of objective circumstances; it requires social endorsement as well.

Undoubtedly some of that endorsement has been afforded by the women's movement, with its persistent emphasis that women's unique needs are apt to be dangerously ignored in social institutions that fail to make gender distinctions. Program development for chronic mentally ill women is emerging in a climate where more general concerns relating to women's health and mental health are increasingly being examined. There have been several landmark publications, including the 1978 report of the subpanel on the mental health of women of the President's Commission on Mental Health (8). In addition, Notman and Nadelson (9–11) have recently edited a three-volume set of papers on women's health and mental health. Both the *American Journal of Psychiatry* (12) and the *American Psychologist* (13) have published special sections of articles on women's mental health issues.

Related publications have addressed the service needs of women who are undomiciled. Baxter and Hopper's classic *Private Lives/Public Spaces* (14) contains a seminal analysis of gender-related differences within the homeless population, many of whose members are overtly and unmistakably mentally ill. An eloquent photo essay by Rousseau (15) graphically supports Baxter and Hopper's narrative. In a report of special hearings on homelessness (16), the United States Congress has reprinted in its entirety an in-depth study of homeless women in Baltimore that pays special attention to those who are mentally ill (17). And in Great Britain, Austerberry and Watson (18) have published a detailed analysis of the housing requirements of homeless women.

Thus, in spite of a paucity of empirical research (19), there is little doubt that awareness of women's gender-related health and mental health issues is growing rapidly in both professional and popular forums.

The specific service problems of chronically mentally ill women are being addressed in this supportive climate, but relative to other gender-related health issues, they have been slow to receive extensive professional attention (20). Test and Berlin (21) have suggested that a lack of professional concern may be related to the fact that the chronic mentally ill are "regarded as almost genderless by both researchers and clinicians." Perhaps this in turn has to do with a deep discomfort that many professionals experience when they confront chronicity. Shulman (22) has observed that "bag ladies," whose severe psychopathology is often apparent and inescapable, remind us uncomfortably of who we might be and what we might become. Ascher (23) has given poetic expression to a similar view in a *New York Times* article. "Whenever I see a bag lady," she has written, "I see myself slipping past the edge of time and space into an abandoned doorway."

Social Legitimation

Blumer (7) wrote that societal recognition originally "gives birth" to a social problem but that if the problem is to "move along on its course and not die aborning," it must become legitimated—that is, it must "acquire social endorsement if it is to be taken seriously and move forward in its career." Program development for chronic mentally ill women similarly requires legitimation before relevant strategies can be implemented.

One method for legitimating social problems is through the appointment of special committees and fact-finding bodies to document specific issues and bring them to public attention. Thus the Michigan Department of Mental Health has named a women's task force that has issued recommendations adverting specifically to the service needs of chronically mentally ill women (24). Similarly, a separate committee on chronic mentally ill women has provided guidance and recommendations to the Women's Mental Health Agenda Conference recently convened by the American Psychological Association in Washington, D.C. (25).

Legitimation also derives from the publication and dissemination of relevant literature. In the case of program development for chronically mentally ill women, a substantial portion of this literature may be found in the popular media. However, in recent years the professional literature has been slowly accumulating and is now beginning to take on a unique identity (20).

Specific Program Issues

The careers of social problems develop at varying speeds and are influenced by such circumstances as the breadth of their bases of support, their ability to demonstrate validity, and the rapidity with which they gain new support. When the social problem is a complex one with many facets, its career may be quite difficult to chart. This is the case with program development for chronic mentally ill women, which consists of a variety of component issues. Some are only emerging; others are already established as bona fide areas of professional interest.

Three specific issues illustrate the composite nature of program development for chronic mentally ill women: homelessness within the population, an issue that is just emerging; skills training, an issue that is maturing and undergoing redefinition; and family planning, an issue that emerged some time ago and has already received substantial legitimation.

Homelessness

Descriptions of the lives and service needs of women who are homeless, disaffiliated, and chronic mentally ill appear regularly in the popular literature. Some of these pieces are sensitive, detailed, and constructive accounts (4, 23, 26–38), and they vastly outnumber reports in the professional literature. And even though professional attention to this issue has recently been increasing (20, 39–41), homelessness among chronic mentally ill women may still be viewed as a newly recognized and emerging concern in program development.

Although it is not possible to provide precise estimates of the proportion of homeless women who are chronically mentally ill (or, for that matter, of the proportion of chronic mentally ill women who are homeless [42]), it is known that the percentage is both marked and rapidly increasing, and that the increase may be attributed largely to the precipitate implementation of deinstitutionalization policies. Thus the population of homeless mentally ill women contains both individuals who have been discharged from institutions and, as the direct consequence of so-called "admission diversion" policies, a growing number who have never been institutionalized at all (43–47).

Evidence exists that homelessness is experienced differently by chronic mentally ill men and women (22, 40). In the first place, it is generally observed—if not actually supported by an empirical data base—that severe psychopathology is more widespread and more intense among homeless women than homeless men. Beyond this,

82

although the provision of shelter is surely inadequate for both sexes, the scarcity of beds is generally considered to be more acute for women than men (14, 40, 48). Baxter and Hopper (14) have graphically described how a shelter in New York City handles this problem by imposing a time limit on the number of nights that women may remain in residence. When they must leave, the women often go directly to train stations or remain on the streets until they are once again eligible for admission.

There are also differences in the social climates of men's and women's shelters. As the result of widespread physical violence, men's shelters are often places where, according to Baxter and Hopper (14), "chronic fear is the rule." But women's shelters tend to be demanding in another sense. They are frequently marked by such excessive regulation and rigidity that pregnant women, women who are drunk or suspected of having used drugs, and those who suffer physical disabilities are denied admission. In fact, a special form of gatekeeping is apparently practiced, at least in New York City (14). Shelter personnel may deny admission to women who have not received psychiatric clearance from Bellevue, a city hospital—a condition not imposed in men's shelters, and one that effectively controls the number of residents by eliminating those women who are fearful of going to Bellevue.

One may speculate on the reasons for such differentials. Are there fewer shelters and more restrictive admission policies for women because women are expected to be responsible for their own domestic arrangements? This puzzling question is in need of analysis. An intriguing exception to the general pattern is provided at the Margaret Frazer House in Toronto, a ten-bed residential facility for chronic mentally ill women (49). Recognizing that members of this population frequently avoid formal intake procedures, staff at Margaret Frazer designate five beds for women referred by hospitals, psychiatric facilities, or social service agencies and reserve the other five beds for women who live on the streets and walk in.

Skills Training

Improving the functional and adaptive skills of chronic mentally ill women is not a new focus in program development, but it is one that is maturing and undergoing redefinition at this time. This evolution is apparent in a change in emphasis in the professional literature within the past decade.

In a 1973 article, for example, Keskiner and his colleagues (50) reported that institutionalized chronic mentally ill women were referred to, accepted by, and placed in foster community programs more readily than were men. The relative ease of placing women was facilitated by different role expectations. Although men were expected to function effectively in outside jobs in order to be placed, women were permitted to assume relatively dependent roles and to be either unemployed or employed in such domestic pursuits as housecleaning and babysitting. Keskiner and his colleagues perceived this differential as advantageous for women and attributed it to the societal role that allows women "greater freedom to express physical and emotional distress and to depend on others for problem solving." Brodsky (51) had reached similar conclusions in an earlier article.

In construing such residential transfer as an index of women's successful deinstitutionalization, Keskiner and his colleagues were using locus of care as their primary outcome criterion. That unemployment or domestic employment might have proved unfulfilling for women who aspired to less stereotyped pursuits and that there might have been quality-of-life considerations exclusive of locational concerns apparently were not considered important in the calculation of advantage.

Although this bias still persists in some program planning for chronic mentally ill women (21, 24), we are at least beginning to assess women's rehabilitative success according to criteria that transcend locus of care and readiness for domestic pursuits. In today's service climate there is more emphasis on preparing chronic mentally ill women to assume a variety of roles in the community, in addition to whatever domestic responsibilities they may undertake (21; Mowbray, C., personal communication, 1985). The role of "meaningful work" in the lives of these patients is increasingly considered critically important to their successful rehabilitation (52).

This is not to say, however, that the preparation of chronic mentally ill women for domestic skills is being abandoned altogether. Indeed, in the areas of parenting and child care, emphasis on effective skills training is actually increasing (21, 24, 53–55). This focus is especially timely because the fertility of chronic mentally ill women is apparently on the rise (56–58). And although it is quite inappropriate to conclude that chronic mentally ill women will necessarily be ineffective mothers (59), there is evidence that some do find motherhood to be particularly stressful—a situation that is likely to have profound implications for their clinical course (60, 61).

Family Planning

Studies of family planning requirements, with related research on sexual functioning and behavior, constitute the best developed portion of the literature on programming for chronic mentally ill women. Family planning is a fully established area of professional concern, with a sophisticated literature and several tested solutions. A variety of topics are subsumed under this general heading, including patients' sexuality; their needs for counseling, sex education, and access to contraceptive methods; and legal and ethical issues related to informed consent (62–72).

This body of work, derived from an ongoing commitment to research and program development, makes it clear that women patients' needs for family planning services increase appreciably in an era of deinstitutionalization. One early study reported a threefold rise in the birth rate of institutionalized women merely as the result of a more liberal policy of leaves and home visits (71). The needs of chronic mentally ill women who are fully resident in the community are undoubtedly even more acute (64).

A parenthetical note that reflects the subtleties of family planning for this population may be added. Talbott and Linn (73) reported in 1978 that many chronic mental patients have atypical perceptions of pain and discomfort, particularly those who experience extended hospital stays. Some simply "lack concern for the physical integrity of their own bodies" and do not respond as expected to pain, physical discomfort, and illness. The implications of this finding for family planning are obvious. Although intrauterine devices might at first glance appear to be the contraceptives of choice for chronic mentally ill women, their use should be considered carefully because of the risk of spontaneous ejection and sequelae of pain and bleeding (64).

Other Issues

As representative aspects of program development for chronic mentally ill women, homelessness, skills training, and family planning illustrate two important points. First, service planning for this population is a complex phenomenon that has a variety of component elements, and, second, each element is itself a discrete planning issue with its own rate of progress. Thus it is probably more meaningful to view program development for this population as a composite phenomenon and not as a unitary event.

Moreover, these three topics must be regarded as illustrative, not exhaustive; other important areas of concern should also be noted. For example, I have discussed elsewhere the unique kinds of stigma that chronic mentally ill women typically endure, and their extreme vulnerability to physical violence and sexual exploitation (20).

Special mention should also be made of concern that exists about the effects of pharmacotherapy on pregnant chronic mentally ill women. Because of its timeliness, this issue will probably achieve legitimation and move toward implementation very rapidly. Toward that end, Nurnberg and Prudic (74) have proposed guidelines to assist psychiatrists in the prescription of psychotropic agents to pregnant women. Similarly, Remick and Maurice (75) have proposed, and Wise and his associates (5) have expanded, guidelines for the safe and efficacious use of ECT during pregnancy.

Concern has also been expressed over neurological side effects of psychotropic agents for nonpregnant women (24, 76). Seeman (77) has found that although schizophrenic women generally respond more favorably to neuroleptics than men, they may complain of weight gain, skin problems, menstrual difficulties, constipation, and pseudopregnancy. Smith and Dunn (78) have reported that women tend to experience a higher prevalence of more severe forms of tardive dyskinesia than men.

Another issue concerns elderly women. Women constitute the major portion of the elderly population in the United States and, similarly, of the elderly chronic mentally ill. They account for more than 70 percent of chronic mentally ill individuals now living in nursing homes (79). Problems specific to treating the elderly chronic mentally ill, such as inappropriate placements and increased mortality risks associated with transfer (4, 80, 81), are therefore largely women's problems.

Still another issue is the admission of chronically mentally ill women needing psychiatric services to jails and correctional facilities. A study by Lamb and Grant (82), unique for its breadth and conceptual clarity, has reported evidence for "diversion into the criminal justice system" of women who before deinstitutionalization "would have been lifetime residents of state hospitals with little chance for possible arrest." In fact, these investigators have documented a constellation of problems characterizing chronically mentally ill women who utilize the criminal justice system, including their inability to find suitable living arrangements, their heavy reliance on prostitution as a means of support, their tendency to engage in crimes of violence, their inability to care for their children, and their lack of access to psychiatric care.

One final important area of concern is the development and implementation of community support systems for chronically mentally ill women. Garrison's work (83) has provided useful insights into network development among Puerto Rican women patients in New York City and has implications for program development for members of other racial and ethnic minority groups. In addition, Segal and Everett-Dille (84) have published data underscoring the importance of social support networks in the development of coping behaviors among chronically mentally ill women.

Comment

A variety of issues are implicit in relevant program planning for chronic mentally ill women, a complex and multifaceted service delivery concern. Some issues are slowly emerging; others have achieved legitimation and endorsement and are moving rapidly toward the proposal and implementation of solutions. The combined effect of these varied efforts has been to bring gender-specific treatment issues for chronic mental patients into clearer focus. This is a positive development, for as Seeman (76) has pointed out, the vicissitudes of chronic mental illness generally differ for men and women, and the "subtleties of gender bear upon all facets of clinical management."

It is important to realize that biological and sociological variables interact in complex ways to create service issues for all chronic mentally ill individuals, men and women alike (85). For example, it has been observed that chronic mentally ill men generally enter the psychiatric service system at younger ages than women (21, 86, 87). The reasons for this differential, and its implications for treatment, require further study. To what extent does women's deferred admission reflect a later onset (76), and to what degree does it indicate that parents or spouses are inclined to "protect" women? Does stereotyping women as "passive, dependent, emotional, and childlike" (8) deprive them of early access to needed psychiatric care?

Beyond this, do sociologically determined expectations serve to bias rehabilitation services for chronic mentally ill women so that they are denied vocational training? As noted above, there is evidence that such a historical bias, so apparent in the program described by Keskiner and his colleagues (50), persists in some places despite efforts to refine outcome assessment criteria (88).

Where such bias does exist, it reflects societal expectations summarized succinctly in a British newspaper article (89). That article notes that if someone asks whether a man should work, the answer is clearly, "'A man *must* work, if he can find a job.' If he can't or loses it and has neither the brains nor the flair to set up on his own, then it is a disaster for his dignity, his self-regard, his manhood even. The whole social order is threatened, not to mention his private domestic one. But if someone asks whether a woman should work, the answer tends to be, 'Yes, OK, if she is unmarried, or if she is childless, or if her children have grown up, or if her husband is unemployed, or if she can fit it in round her other responsibilities to the family....' If, if, if. Or, or, or. It is somehow always seen as a choice, a dilemma, an *option*.'

Thus rehabilitation programs for chronic mentally ill men are more likely to be based on higher expectations of performance than are programs for women, in possible contravention of clinical precepts (90). The hope that chronic mentally ill men will eventually become economically productive citizens, and the expectation that women will not, generates different patterns of placement in deinstitutionalized service systems and different emphases in treatment planning. It may even have profound effects on program areas that are not specifically vocational, such as housing, and thus contribute in some way to homelessness among chronic mentally ill women.

This situation leads to the conclusion that when treatment proceeds on the basis of gender stereotypes instead of individual patients' needs, it may be manifestly harmful to chronic mentally ill men as well as women. Once again, divergent vocational role expectations may be used to illustrate the point. Chronic mentally ill individuals often have problems in tolerating stress (61), and from this perspective it is possible that a man will have more difficulty than a woman in finding a stress-free environment in the community. Indeed, to some extent a woman's home may provide her with a "sheltered workshop" (91) that can insulate her and give her needed asylum (51, 92). A man, by contrast, may well find little relief from unrealistically high expectations, particularly in the area of employment (93, 94).

Finally, as noted previously, the women's movement has undoubtedly played a critical role in hastening the emergence of specialized programming for chronic mentally ill women. A debt of gratitude for that assistance is due. At the same time, however, it is important to understand that whenever social or health issues emerge in a political context, there is a risk of unnecessary politicization and, perhaps, of unwarranted penalty.

A most dramatic example has occurred in California, where Roman Catholic social workers in Los Angeles County have been ordered to stop referring homeless women to a shelter operated by a nun with a reported "proabortion position" (95). Although some might question the rational justification for such a move, the fact that it has even occurred holds a lesson for those who attempt to implement policy in the midst of political controversy. Care must be taken to avoid confounding issues with extraneous variables.

The emergence and legitimation of program issues for chronic mentally ill women may be viewed as a positive step in the refinement of services for people who suffer from chronic mental illnesses. As specific issues in service delivery come to the fore, are realistically assessed, and move toward relevant solutions, we may anticipate a sharpening of planning concepts. This in turn should lead to more appropriate service planning for a population whose needs are frequently overlooked. We may expect that in such a climate the requirements of chronic mentally ill women—and also of chronically mentally ill men—will be more sensitively met.

References

1. Evans S, Lewis AE: Woman, 86, freezes to death. Washington Post, 17 January 1985, p 12
2. Evans S: Freezing death angers SE church. Washington Post, 19 January 1985, p D2
3. McLaughlin L: Mental health center death being probed. Boston Globe, 11 December 1984, pp 1,6
4. Carmody D: The tangled life and mind of Judy, whose home is the street. New York Times, 17 December 1984, pp B1, B10
5. Wise MG, Ward SC, Townsend-Parchman W, et al: Case report of ECT during high-risk pregnancy. Am J Psychiatry 141:99–101, 1984
6. Lovejoy M: Recovery from Schizophrenia: a personal odyssey. Hosp Community Psychiatry 35:809–812, 1984
7. Blumer H: Social problems as collective behavior. Social Problems 18:298–306, 1971
8. President's Commission on Mental Health: Report of the Subpanel on the Mental Health of Women, in Report to the President, vol 3. Washington, DC, US Government Printing Office, 1978
9. Notman MT, Nadelson CC (eds): The Woman Patient, vol 1. Sexual and Reproductive Aspects of Women's Health Care. New York, Plenum, 1978
10. Nadelson CC, Notman MT (eds): The Woman Patient, vol 2. Concepts of Femininity and the Life Cycle. New York, Plenum, 1982
11. Notman MT, Nadelson CC (eds): The Woman Patient, vol 3. Aggression, Adaptations, and Psychotherapy. New York, Plenum, 1982
12. Special section: personal and professional issues for women. Am J Psychiatry 138: 1317–1361, 1981
13. Women, psychology, and public policy: selected issues. Am Psychol 39:1161–1192, 1984
14. Baxter E, Hopper K: Private Lives/Public Spaces: Homeless Adults on the Streets of New York City. New York, Community Service Society, 1981
15. Rousseau AM: Shopping Bag Ladies. New York, Pilgrim Press, 1981

16. Hearing Before the Subcommittee on Housing and Community Development, US Congress, 15 December 1982. Serial no. 97–100. Washington, DC, US Government Printing Office, 1983
17. Walsh B, Davenport D: The Long Loneliness in Baltimore: A Study of Homeless Women. Baltimore, Viva House, 1981
18. Austerberry H, Watson S: Women on the Margins: A Study of Single Women's Housing Problems. London, City University Housing Research Group, 1983
19. Carmen E, Russo NF, Miller JB: Inequality and women's mental health: an overview. Am J Psychiatry 138:1319–1330, 1981
20. Bachrach LL: Deinstitutionalization and women: assessing the consequences of public policy. Am Psychol 39:1171–1177, 1984
21. Test MA, Berlin SB: Issues of special concern to chronically mentally ill women. Professional Psychology 12:136–145, 1981
22. Shulman AK: Preface, in Shopping Bag Ladies, by Rousseau AM. New York, Pilgrim Press, 1981
23. Ascher BL: Hers. New York Times, 17 February 1983, p C2
24. Women's Task Force: For Better or Worse? Women and the Mental Health System. Lansing, Michigan Department of Mental Health, April 1982
25. Report From the National Women's Mental Health Agenda Conference. Washington, DC, American Psychological Association, January 1985
26. Bassuk E: Addressing the needs of the homeless. Boston Globe Magazine, 6 November 1983, pp 12, 60ff
27. Campbell BM: We're learning to harden our hearts and shrug our shoulders. Washington Post, 26 December 1982, pp D1, D4
28. Gilliam D: Bag-lady chic. Washington Post, 9 July 1983, p B1
29. Kaplan JL: Homeless, hungry, and Jewish. Washington Jewish Week, 16 February 1984, pp 1, 4–5
30. Krucoff C: Psychiatrist of the streets. Washington Post, 24 May 1984, pp D1, D15
31. McCarthy C: The "bag ladies": there's no place like homeless. Washington Post, 7 November 1982, pp B1, B2
32. Overend W: The LA bag lady who chose to be one. Los Angeles Times, 16 July 1983, pp 1, 4
33. Overend W: What can be done about Laura Juarez? Los Angeles Times, 9 October 1983, pp 1, 16–18
34. Peters JW: Women also tread path to confinement. Evening Sun (Baltimore), 28 August 1984, pp A1, A4

35. Quindlen A: Despite frigid weather, many homeless women still shun shelters. New York Times, 15 December 1982, p B3
36. Torrey EF: The real twilight zone. Washington Post, 26 August 1983, p A9
37. White RD: On the streets. Washington Post, 22 January 1985, p A19
38. Zibart E: A wispy life. Washington Post, 8 December 1983, p Md1
39. Crystal S: Homeless men and women: the gender gap. Urban and Social Change Review 17(Summer):2–6, 1984
40. Schwam K: Shopping Bag Ladies: Homeless Women. New York, Manhattan Bowery Corporation, 1979
41. Slavinsky AT, Cousins A: Homeless women. Nurs Outlook 30:358–362, 1982
42. Bachrach LL: Interpreting research on the homeless mentally ill: some caveats. Hosp Community Psychiatry 35:914–917, 1984
43. Dionne EJ: Mental patient cutbacks planned. New York Times, 8 December 1978, p B3
44. Morrissey JP, McGreevy MM: The fates of applicants denied admission to state mental hospitals: some unexpected consequences of deinstitutionalization in the USA. Presented at the meeting of the International Sociological Association, Mexico City, August 1981
45. Pepper B, Ryglewicz H: Testimony for the neglected: the mentally ill in the post-deinstitutionalized age. Am J Orthopsychiatry 52:388–391, 1982
46. Shapiro JG: Patients refused admission to a psychiatric hospital. Hosp Community Psychiatry 34:733–736, 1983
47. Sullivan R: Hospital forced to oust patients with psychoses. New York Times, 8 November 1979, p A1
48. Recovery not felt in Houston. Safety Network (newsletter, National Coalition for the Homeless, New York City), January 1985, pp 2–3
49. Information for Referring Sources. Toronto, Margaret Frazer House, 1984
50. Keskiner A, Zalcman MJ, Ruppert EH: Advantages of being female in psychiatric rehabilitation. Arch Gen Psychiatry 28:689–692, 1973

51. Brodsky CM: The social recovery of mentally ill housewives. Fam Process 7:170–183, 1968

52. Houghton J: On personal experience: before and after mental illness, in Attitudes Toward the Mentally Ill: Research Perspectives. Edited by Rabkin JG, Gelb L, Lazar JB. Rockville, MD, National Institute of Mental Health, 1980

53. Gochman ERG, Aisenstein C: Preventive Therapy With High-Risk Mothers by the Mother and Infant Development Program, Washington, DC, St. Elizabeths Hospital, April 1983

54. Parry C: Domestic roles, in Theory and Practice of Psychiatric Rehabilitation. Edited by Watts FN, Bennett DH. Chichester, England, Wiley, 1983

55. Gold award: a treatment and education program for emotionally disturbed women and their young children. Hosp Community Psychiatry 31:687–689, 1980

56. APA award honors Providence Center. National Council of Community Mental Health Centers News, November 1984, pp 6, 14

57. Pepper B, Ryglewicz H: Treating the young adult chronic patient: an update. New Directions for Mental Health Services, no. 21, pp 5–15, 1984

58. Test MA, Knoedler WH, Allness DJ, et al: Young adults with schizophrenic disorders in the community. Presented at the annual meeting of the American Psychiatric Association, Los Angeles, 5–11 May, 1984

59. Poole SR, Sharer DR, Barbee MA, et al: Hospitalization of a psychotic mother and her breast-feeding infant. Hosp Community Psychiatry 31:412–414, 1980

60. Keitner C, Grof P: Sexual and emotional intimacy between psychiatric inpatients; formulating a policy. Hosp Community Psychiatry 32:188–193, 1981

61. Lamb HR: Treating the Long-Term Mentally Ill: Beyond Deinstitutionalization. San Francisco, Jossey-Bass, 1982

62. Abernethy V: Sexual knowledge, attitudes, and practices of young female psychiatric patients. Arch Gen Psychiatry 30:180–182, 1974

63. Abernethy V, Grunebaum H: Family planning in two psychiatric hospitals: a preliminary report. Fam Plann Perspect 5:94–99, 1973

64. Abernethy V, Grunebaum H, Clough L, et al: Family planning during psychiatric hospitalization. Am J Orthopsychiatry 46:154–162, 1976

65. Clough L, Abernethy V, Grunebaum H: Contraception for the severely psychiatrically disturbed: confusion, control, and contraindication. Compr Psychiatry 17:601–606, 1976

66. Grunebaum H, Abernethy V: Ethical issues in family planning for hospitalized psychiatric patients. Am J Psychiatry 132:236–240, 1975

67. Grunebaum HU, Abernethy VD, Rofman ES, et al: The family planning attitudes, practices, and motivations of mental patients. Am J Psychiatry 128:740–744, 1971

68. Lyketsos GC, Sakka P, Mailis A: The sexual adjustment of chronic schizophrenics: a preliminary study. Br J Psychiatry 143:376–382, 1983

69. McEvoy JP, Hatcher A, Appelbaum PS, et al: Chronic schizophrenic women's attitudes toward sex, pregnancy, birth control, and childrearing. Hosp Community Psychiatry 34:536–539, 1983

70. Rozensky RH, Berman C: Sexual knowledge, attitudes, and experiences of chronic psychiatric patients. Psychosocial Rehabilitation Journal 8:21–27, 1984

71. Shearer ML, Cain AC, Finch SM, et al: Unexpected effects of an "open door" policy on birth rates of women in state hospitals. Am J Orthopsychiatry 38:413–417, 1968

72. Verhulst J, Schneidman B: Schizophrenia and sexual functioning. Hosp Community Psychiatry 32:259–262, 1981

73. Talbott JA, Linn L: Reactions of schizophrenics to life-threatening disease. Psychiatric Q 50:218–227, 1978

74. Nurnberg HG, Prudic J: Guidelines for treatment of psychosis during pregnancy. Hosp Community Psychiatry 35:67–71, 1984

75. Remick RA, Maurice WL: ECT in pregnancy (letter). Am J Psychiatry 135:761–762, 1978

76. Seeman MV: Schizophrenic men and women require different treatment programs. Journal of Psychiatric Treatment and Evaluation 5:143–148, 1983

77. Seeman MV: Gender differences in schizophrenia. Can J Psychiatry 27:107–112, 1982

78. Smith JM, Dunn DD: Sex differences in the prevalence of severe tardive dyskinesia. Am J Psychiatry 136:1080–1083, 1979

79. Cicchinelli LF, Bell JC, Dittmar ND, et al: Factors Influencing the Deinstitutionalization of the Mentally Ill: A Review and Analysis. Denver, Denver Research Institute, 1981
80. Black DW, Warrack G, Winokur G: Excess mortality among psychiatric patients. JAMA 253:58–61, 1985
81. Marlowe RA: When they closed the door at Modesto, in Where Is My Home? Proceedings of a Conference on the Closing of State Mental Hospitals. Menlo Park, CA, Stanford Research Institute, 1974
82. Lamb HR, Grant RW: Mentally ill women in a county jail. Arch Gen Psychiatry 40:363–368, 1983
83. Garrison V: Support systems of schizophrenic and nonschizophrenic Puerto Rican migrant women in New York City. Schizophrenia Bull 4:561–596, 1978
84. Segal SP, Everett-Dille L: Coping styles and factors in male/female social integration. Acta Psychiatr Scand 61:8–20, 1980
85. Mechanic D: Sex, illness behavior, and the use of health services. Social Sci Med 12B:207–214, 1978
86. Knoedler W: Persons With Chronic Mental Illness and CSP. Madison, Wisc, CSP Information Exchange, Wisconsin Department of Health and Social Services, April 1984
87. Lewine RRJ: Sex differences in age of symptom onset and first hospitalization in schizophrenia. Am J Orthopsychiatry 50:316–322, 1980
88. Bachrach LL: Assessment of outcomes in community support systems: results, problems, and limitations. Schizophrenia Bull 8:39–61, 1982
89. Lowry S: The woman executive is as androgynous as Boy George. The Guardian (London), 20 September 1984, p 19
90. Test MA, Stein LI: Special living arrangements: a model for decision-making. Hosp Community Psychiatry 28:608–610, 1977
91. Tudor W, Tudor JF, Gove WR: The effect of sex role differences on the social control of mental illness. J Health Soc Behav 18:98–112, 1977
92. Bachrach LL: Asylum and chronically ill psychiatric patients. Am J Psychiatry 141:975–978, 1984
93. Huffine CL, Clausen JA: Madness and work: short- and long-term effects of mental illness on occupational careers. Social Forces 57:1049–1062, 1979

94. Kinard EM, Klerman LV: Changes in life style following mental hospitalization. J Nerv Ment Dis 168:666–672, 1980
95. Shelter is ruled off-limits. Washington Post, 25 January 1985, p A8

Deferred Pelvic Examinations: A Purposeful Omission in the Care of Mentally Ill Women

MARYELLEN H. HANDEL, Ph.D.

Deferred Pelvic Examinations: A Purposeful Omission in the Care of Mentally Ill Women

In their struggle to meet the multiple psychiatric and rehabilitative needs of the many chronic mentally ill living in the community, community mental health centers and aftercare clinics have overlooked the importance of pelvic examinations for women patients. The author presents a review of the literature focusing on the reasons that such exams are generally deferred and the arguments that support conducting complete physical examinations of women psychiatric patients. She then presents results of a study that indicate the extent to which pelvic examinations are deferred, suggests steps that facilities can take to rectify the problem, and poses questions for further research.

*T*he chronically ill woman psychiatric patient presents mental health providers with a host of special problems (1–3). The mandate to provide comprehensive medical treatment and monitoring for the chronically disabled (4) should explicitly include attention to gynecological issues. Clearly, many women in the general population lack comprehensive gynecological care. However, for deinstitutionalized females, additional factors serve to prevent easy access to this essential aspect of ongoing care.

Although the medical care of psychiatric patients has been a continuing concern (5–16), few articles in the literature focus on the deinstitutionalized patient, and none are specifically devoted to the gynecological treatment of the chronically ill woman who lives in the community. Because community mental health centers and aftercare clinics must struggle to coordinate services for the multiple psychiatric and rehabilitative needs of the chronically ill (17), they may overlook the medical needs of these patients.

Often the centers and clinics monitor the physical health of the deinstitutionalized population through records of the medical examinations carried out in emergency rooms and inpatient psychiatric services. However, it is not possible to rely on these examinations to adequately meet the gynecological health needs of women psychiatric patients, for it is standard practice in both emergency rooms and inpatient psychiatric units to omit the pelvic examination and to state on the patient's record that the exam has been "deferred."

Reasons for Deferring Pelvic Examinations

Many reasons are given for deferring pelvic examinations for mentally ill women.

The chronic mentally ill are seen as genderless

Many authors (2, 18) point out that patients with major mental illnesses are not viewed by caregivers, researchers, or policymakers as having specific needs based on their gender. A widely held attitude has been that "the problems related to the illness are so massive that there just isn't time or energy to think about [the patients] as women or men" (1). Test and Berlin (1) state that "lack of attention to gender-related issues of the chronic mentally ill has hampered knowledge and understanding of these persons' disorders as well as compounded their problems in daily living." Researchers and clinicians (1–3, 18) are beginning to look at the particular social and psychiatric needs of chronically ill women, but as yet guidelines for the medical care of mentally ill women have not been specifically addressed in clinical settings.

Once an individual is labeled a psychiatric patient, his or her physical problems may be overlooked

In a study of diagnostic errors in the evaluation of psychiatric patients in the emergency room setting, Leeman (11) found that if the evaluators focused on the patient's psychological status or social setting, they might not pursue physical factors. In many cases psychiatric patients present with a mixed clinical picture of physical as well as emotional problems. However, once a patient is given a psychiatric diagnosis, the evaluators generally do not look for a physical problem. Therefore, when the patient is a female with major mental illness, it becomes even less likely that a pelvic examination will be carried out.

The chronically ill may be unable to give clear indications of locus of pain

If a patient complains of abdominal pain, it is more likely that a pelvic examination will be carried out. However, Talbott and Linn (19) have pointed out that the severely mentally ill differ in their ability to communicate about pain or discomfort. Reporting a study of medically ill psychiatric patients in state facilities, they noted that the "most striking and pervasive finding was that many psychotic patients with severe and dramatic illnesses, which produce pain in most patients, verbalized no discomfort" (19). If women with major mental illness are not able to communicate physical symptoms such as abdominal pain, pelvic examinations may be deferred.

Psychiatrists may believe that carrying out a pelvic examination will interfere with the patient-therapist relationship

In hospital settings where psychiatric residents may perform the physical examination of female patients whom they may later treat in psychotherapy, transference and countertransference concerns are important. Psychiatrists often believe that performing the physical examination is detrimental to the psychotherapeutic relationship (12). Some, however, have suggested that it may be useful (12, 14). If a psychiatrist has doubts about performing a physical examination, carrying one out will certainly be problematic.

Physicians may fear malpractice suits

In a study of the attitudes of psychiatric residents, psychiatrists, internists, and fourth-year medical students about performing physical examinations of psychiatric patients, McIntyre and Romano

(12) found that all four groups frequently omitted the pelvic examination. After surveying the respondents about this omission, the authors concluded that it is not the clinical, cognitive, or emotional state(s) of the patient that account for the omission." Rather, especially for the psychiatrists, the threat of malpractice suits may underlie the decision to omit the pelvic examination.

Although McIntyre and Romano believe the risk of possible law suits is minimal, they and others (20) suggest that psychiatric practitioners use chaperones when examining patients and seek consultation with other specialists when necessary. When male psychiatrists are responsible for carrying out physical examinations of female patients, the pelvic examination may be omitted on the slim chance of possible litigation.

Psychiatric staff may not feel able to perform physical examinations

The physical examination in a psychiatric setting may be carried out by psychiatric residents or psychiatrists who do not feel competent to carry out a pelvic examination. Because of specialization in training, psychiatrists are rarely asked to perform a physical examination after residency. As the years separating training from practice increase, confidence in carrying out the examination decreases (21, 22).

A significant percentage of psychiatrists in McIntyre and Romano's study (12) stated that they did not carry out physical examinations because they did not feel competent to do so. Patterson's survey (22) of 98 psychiatrists indicated that 53 percent gave "no longer feel competent" as the reason for not performing routine physical examinations.

Because of the reasons discussed, it is not surprising that deferral of the pelvic examination has become standard for mentally ill women. Yet this omission profoundly affects the overall health care of the deinstitutionalized woman patient.

Reasons for Performing Pelvic Examinations

The pelvic examination should be an integral part of the medical evaluation of the mentally ill woman for several reasons.

102

Psychiatric populations have a high incidence of physical illness

Comprehensive medical examinations of psychiatric patients are essential because of the high incidence of physical illness among this population (7-10, 14-16). Researchers examining psychiatric populations specifically for physical illness have found positive results in 33 to 60 percent of the patients (6, 8, 12). Many of these illnesses have been previously undetected by either the patient or his or her physician (6, 16). Findings indicate that cardiovascular and endocrine problems are most frequently implicated (6).

Hall and colleagues (6) carried out comprehensive physical examinations of 55 psychiatric women patients and found that 2 had precancerous conditions (a positive stage II Pap smear and multiple vaginal polyps) that required surgery. Weingarten and colleagues' (16) evaluation of a group of geropsychiatric patients found that 22 percent of the women had gynecological problems. The following case exemplifies the problem.

A physician was asked to assess a mentally ill woman who came to the emergency room with vague physical complaints in the area of the neck and upper torso. A physical evaluation revealed no significant findings, and the patient was to be sent home.

However, the family members who accompanied the patient insisted that something was wrong, and the physician completed the physical evaluation by carrying out a pelvic examination. An advanced malignant uterine tumor was found and subsequently treated surgically. Had the patient been alone, the pelvic examination would not have been performed.

The community system of treatment delivery is not comprehensive

The deinstitutionalization process has created a myriad of services provided by various community agencies (17). Thus patients may be seen in a variety of settings, and their records may be scattered with no continuously reliable data base available for clinical evaluators.

This situation contrasts with the large state hospital system of the past, which kept medical records for years. Periodic physical evaluations could be carried out according to established clinical protocols (10). For patients in this system, diagnostic evaluations might be performed in response to staff who saw the patient daily and who observed some abnormality or alteration in their emotional state (19).

In the absence of a truly comprehensive system of treatment delivery, the standardization of a gynecological examination in inpatient units and aftercare clinics would help assure that the physical well-being of female patients living in the community is not being overlooked. Talbott and Linn (19) have stated that the current trend toward ambulatory, community-based treatment for chronic mental patients raises concerns that serious medical conditions might go unnoticed.

Women patients perceive the pelvic examination to be important for their medical care

A recent survey asked 69 female psychiatric patients at a Veterans Administration facility about their satisfaction with the services they received and also about the types of services they would like to have provided (23). Respondents were asked to rank-order their preferences. Requests for pelvic examinations and Pap smears were ranked second after instruction in breast self-examination. As a result of this study, procedural guidelines have been implemented to ensure that pelvic examinations are performed as part of the routine physical examinations on the inpatient units of this facility (23).

The pelvic examination may be lifesaving

Because psychiatric patients may be prelabeled, their physical complaints may be unheeded and attributed to emotional problems (11). The chronic woman patient living in the community may be at risk if she has no advocate and tries to gain medical help for gynecological problems. Life-threatening conditions that can be properly diagnosed only through a pelvic examination may go undetected because of the frequent decision of evaluating physicians to defer examination. Two case examples vividly dramatize this point.

Case 1. Koranyi (9) reports the case of a 24-year-old schizophrenic woman who died of peritonitis, internal bleeding, and aspiration of gastric contents following perforation by her intrauterine device. She had complained of intense lower abdominal pain for several weeks before her death, had visited the emergency room of a local general hospital on several occasions, and had been repeatedly told that her condition was "psychosomatic."

Case 2. While in a seclusion room of a mental health center, a 27-year-old woman with a history of psychiatric hospitalizations bled to death because of an undetected ruptured tubal pregnancy. When she first sought emergency care for abdominal pain at a general hospital, she was referred to another emergency room for admission to the inpatient unit of the mental health center, where she died two days later (24).

In both these cases, a pelvic examination was medically indicated and, properly performed, might have avoided these fatalities. Both women were chronically mentally ill with few resources. One lived in shelters but was often homeless. Both may be typical of the chronically ill deinstitutionalized women who are at greatest risk. If we are to "focus our attention on the patients we have responsibility for treating," a closer look at the deferred pelvic examination for chronic psychiatric patients is certainly indicated (25).

How Extensive Is the Problem?

To ascertain the extent of deferred pelvic examinations in our area, we studied the psychiatric hospital admissions from our aftercare service from October 1983 through September 1984. The aftercare service is located in a suburb of Boston and had a roster of 120 patients, 64 of whom were female.

During the study, 24 women were hospitalized. Ninety percent were admitted to the inpatient units in a community hospital and 10 percent to a state facility. Review of physical examinations performed at admission on these patients indicated omission of the pelvic examination in every case.

To ascertain whether the 24 female aftercare patients were typical in not having received pelvic examinations, we also surveyed all the female admissions to both the state hospital and the general hospital psychiatric units during 1984. In that year the state hospital facility had 35 female admissions, and in each case the pelvic examination was deferred. The psychiatric units of the general hospital had 416 female admissions and, as a matter of course, the pelvic examinations were omitted on initial physical examination.

A consistent pattern of omitted pelvic examinations is apparent in this particular, yet not atypical, catchment area. Although deinstitutionalized women patients require gynecological examinations for health maintenance, we found that this is not a standard procedure when they are hospitalized.

Implications for Health Care Policy

The literature survey and our small study underscore a problem in the delivery of comprehensive treatment to chronic mentally ill women. It appears clear that complete physical examinations, including pelvic examinations, should be provided for all psychiatric patients but have been omitted in many cases.

To ameliorate this problem, psychiatric facilities must first make a commitment to carry out a complete physical examination for all patients. For women patients, this would include a complete gynecological-obstetric history; a pelvic, abdominal, and breast examination; and a Pap smear (26). For male patients, the physical would include a rectal examination and an examination for testicular cancer detection. The conviction that all psychiatric patients require and will receive a comprehensive medical examination must lie at the heart of any treatment policies.

Next, health care agencies must specify who will carry out pelvic examinations on a routine basis. If psychiatrists are to perform this function, they must feel competent to do so. Retraining and continued education must be provided for staff who have lost this skill.

However, consulting gynecological staff, nurse practitioners, or other nonpsychiatric medical personnel might routinely conduct a gynecological evaluation of patients upon admission to psychiatric inpatient units and aftercare clinics. The gynecological care of the patient would still be deemed an essential aspect of care but would be considered a specialty like the routine ocular or dental consultation.

Third, problems involving space may have to be solved. Adequate space may be a problem for psychiatric inpatient units and outpatient agencies that do not now require pelvic examinations for female patients. In addition, many inpatient psychiatric units have small treatment rooms that are poorly equipped for carrying out pelvic examinations. If psychiatric facilities make the commitment to routinely conduct a complete gynecological examination of women patients and carry out Pap smears, the appropriate space and equipment must be provided.

Finally, staff must consider the patient's mental status before performing pelvic examinations. Certainly, if patients are floridly psychotic and not able to cooperate with the examiner, only a limited physical examination can be performed (20). However, facilities can still require staff to document and follow up on a patient's physical condition until the complete examination has been performed. Whenever possible, the physical complaints of a patient in distress should be immediately addressed. In all cases, policies should be based on standards of excellence for both the psychiatric and the medical care of the patient.

Research Directions

The low priority given the gynecological care of female deinstitutionalized patients has not only put them at risk but has created a gap in our knowledge of this population. As pelvic examinations become routine, a baseline for gathering data will be established.

Further research should answer some of the following questions:

1. How universal are deferred pelvic examinations?
2. What is the extent of gynecological problems in various populations of mentally ill women? How do such populations compare with normal controls?
3. Who should carry out pelvic examinations in inpatient units, in day hospital programs, and in outpatient clinics?
4. What are the gynecological health care needs of mentally ill women? What educational programs need to be instituted to enhance health maintenance? Are resources available in the community to meet these needs?
5. How can emergency room staff become more alert to the need for gynecological evaluation of mentally ill women?
6. Which subgroups of mentally ill women are more at risk for gynecological problems? How can we ensure that their needs are more adequately met?

Conclusion

The practice of omitting pelvic examinations for psychiatric patients is but one example of how the most basic health care needs of the chronically ill are overlooked. The task of providing for the psychiatric, social, and rehabilitative needs of deinstitutionalized patients is massive. Yet evidence indicates that a focus on the medical care of the mentally ill patient is also essential.

The problem of the deferred pelvic examination highlights in particular the manner in which specific gender-related treatments have been ignored. Further research and implementation of policies that value the overall health care of the chronically mentally ill woman are certainly indicated.

References

1. Test MA, Berlin S: Issues of special concern to chronically mentally ill women. Professional Psychology 12:136–145, 1981
2. Bachrach LL: Deinstitutionalization and women: assessing the consequences of public policy. Am Psychol 39:1171–1177, 1984
3. Seeman MV: Schizophrenic men and women require different treatment programs. Journal of Psychiatric Treatment and Evaluation 5:143–148, 1983
4. Bachrach LL: Asylum and chronically ill psychiatric patients. Am J Psychiatry 141:975–978, 1984
5. Anath J: Physical illness and psychiatric disorder. Compr Psychiatry 25:586–593, 1984
6. Hall RC, Gardner ER, Stickney SK, et al: Physical illness manifesting as psychiatric disease. II. Analysis of a state hospital inpatient population. Arch Gen Psychiatry 37:989–995, 1980
7. Johnson DAW: The evaluation of routine physical examinations in psychiatric cases. Practitioner 200:686–691, 1968
8. Karasu TB, Waltzman SA, Lindenmayer JP, et al: The medical care of patients with psychiatric illness. Hosp Community Psychiatry 31:463–472, 1980
9. Koranyi EK: Fatalities in 2,070 psychiatric outpatients: preventative features. Arch Gen Psychiatry 34:1137–1142, 1977
10. Lansbury J: The prevalence of physical disease in a large mental hospital and its implications for staffing. Hosp Community Psychiatry 23:148–151, 1972

11. Leeman C: Diagnostic errors in emergency room medicine: physical illness in patients labeled "psychiatric" and vice versa. Int J Psychiatry Med 6:533–540, 1975
12. McIntyre JS, Romano J: Is there a stethoscope in the house (and is it used)? Arch Gen Psychiatry 34:1147–1151, 1977
13. Mannino FV, Wylie HW: Evaluation of the physical examination as part of psychiatric clinic intake practice. Am J Psychiatry 122:175–179, 1965
14. Summers WK, Munoz RA, Read MR: The psychiatric physical examination, part I: methodology. J Clin Psychiatry 42:95–98, 1981
15. Summers WK, Munoz RA, Read MR, et al: The psychiatric physical examination, part II: findings in 75 unselected psychiatric patients. J Clin Psychiatry 42:99–102, 1981
16. Weingarten CH, Rosoff LG, Eisen SV, et al: Medical care in a geriatric psychiatry unit: impact on psychiatric outcome. J Am Geriatr Soc 30:738–742, 1982
17. Bachrach LL: Continuity of care for chronic mental patients: a conceptual analysis. Am J Psychiatry 138:1449–1456, 1981
18. Carmen E, Russo NF, Miller JB: Inequality and women's mental health: an overview. Am J Psychiatry 138:1319–1330, 1981
19. Talbott JA, Linn L: Reactions of schizophrenics to life-threatening disease. Psychiatric Q 50:218–227, 1978
20. Menninger KA, Mayman M, Pruyser PW: A Manual for Psychiatric Case Study, 2nd ed. New York, Grune & Stratton, 1962
21. Liptzin B: Psychiatrists are also physicians. Arch Gen Psychiatry 39:113–114, 1982
22. Patterson CW: Psychiatrists and physical examinations: a survey. Am J Psychiatry 135:967–968, 1978
23. Rothman GH: Needs of female patients in a veterans psychiatric hospital. Social Work 29:380–385, 1984
24. McLaughlin L: Mental health center death being probed. Boston Globe, 11 December 1984, pp. 1, 6
25. Talbott JA: Response to the presidential address: psychiatry's unfinished business in the 20th century. Am J Psychiatry 141:927–930, 1984
26. McBurney RD: Gynecologic care at a state hospital for the mentally ill. Am J Obstet Gynecol 95:345–349, 1966

Chapter 8

Development of a Program to Improve the Care of Chronically Mentally Ill Women

MARYELLEN H. HANDEL, Ph.D.
MONA BLEIBERG BENNETT, M.D.

Chapter 8

Development of a Program to Improve the Care of Chronically Mentally Ill Women

The material contained in this chapter grew out of the research described in Chapter 7. The authors emphasize program implementation related to gender-specific issues. They highlight the need for attention to similarities and differences in the symptoms, course of illness, and treatment requirements for men and women and point to the need for collaborative efforts. They focus specifically on collaboration with the specialty of obstetrics and gynecology to provide a full range of medical services for chronically mentally ill women.

*T*here are three important components to consider in planning and implementing new programs for chronically mentally ill women: assessing standard data in new ways; introducing new initiatives based on needs highlighted by research; and evaluating those initiatives to ascertain whether they have fulfilled the needs brought to light by the research.

This chapter addresses the second component, the program implementation stage. First, we discuss the importance of actuating policies that respond to gender-specific needs among the chronically mentally ill and describe the administrative environment in which such program planning presently occurs. Then we present a case history to illustrate how one administrator implemented a public health program for chronically mentally ill women. Finally, we attempt to draw some conclusions from our experience that may help others who seek to implement new interventions for chronically mentally ill inpatients in a general hospital setting.

Importance of Gender-Specific Planning

In the last decade, there has been a growing awareness of both the need for continuity of care for chronic mental patients (1–4) and the existence of a variety of subpopulations whose specific treatment needs differ. Thus, Bachrach (1) writes, "Planning for continuity of care must always start with the most basic question: Are all persons in the planning universe being considered, or is some portion of that universe experiencing discrimination? Continuity of care will vary according to the needs of different subpopulations of the chronically mentally ill, and our planning should reflect this fact" (1).

The specific importance of gender differences within the chronically mentally ill population has also been documented in recent years (5–7), and the psychiatric literature has now clearly designated chronically mentally ill women as a critical subgroup with specific needs and particular clinical presentations. Women who are mentally ill may present a very different clinical picture from that presented by mentally ill men (8–10). In addition, there are indications that gender differences within the chronically mentally ill population, and their medical, social, and family planning implications, must no longer be ignored if high-quality care is to be afforded the chronically mentally ill (5–7, 11–14).

In light of these findings, it is apparent that innovative programs that respect the unique needs of all chronically mentally ill individuals must not regard the male patient as the sole point of departure in program planning. Program needs that specifically apply to female patients must also be respected. It follows that, if we make a conscious effort to address issues of gender, we shall have moved toward fulfilling the mandate for continuity of care and toward establishing an overall therapeutic holding environment for mentally ill individuals in the community.

Once the administrator has looked at the needs of the chronically mentally ill in this new way, it is then his or her obligation to translate this perspective into relevant policies and programs for treatment. As Granet and Talbott (3) point out, "the failure to achieve continuity of care does not result so much from a lack of knowledge about how to deal with chronic patients as it does from a *failure to apply what we know*" [emphasis added].

However, a number of difficulties are associated with applying what we know about gender-specific inequalities in the planning of

114

programs for chronically mentally ill individuals in today's service systems, and many of these are administrative in nature. These difficulties must be analyzed and addressed.

The Administrative Environment

During the 1960s and 1970s the planning imperative for the mental health administrator was to move patients from institutional custodial care settings into the community and into more active treatment (15). By contrast, the administrative goal for mental health care in the 1980s is to provide equal access to services, assessment procedures, treatment programs, and continuity of care for all chronic mental patients, wherever they are. This mandate calls for the administrator to balance the needs of specific subgroups—such as women, men, racial and ethnic minorities, neurologically damaged individuals, and adolescents—within the chronically mentally ill population. This balance must be established in a time of cost-cutting, shrinking resources, and diminishing federal support (16, 17).

Thus, the administrator who wishes to respond to gender-specific treatment needs within the chronically mentally ill patient population must work out a strategy of implementation that fits in with contemporary administrative realities. In so doing he or she must organize a plan that both supports state-of-the-art technologies in the care of chronic mental patients and also responds to administrative realities. This process is achieved by following a series of steps: 1) initiating program plans for chronically mentally ill women on the basis of current research findings; 2) anticipating and planning for probable resistances to change; 3) responding actively to the challenge of external barriers; 4) deliberating and weighing conflicting interests; and 5) implementing the new program. After these steps have been completed, the administrator must then proceed to monitor the new program's effectiveness through evaluative research.

The following case study relates a series of events that ensued at the Newton-Wellesley Hospital, a university-affiliated general hospital in a suburb of Boston, when the Department of Psychiatry, following the steps outlined above, established a program responding to the gynecological health care needs of chronically mentally ill women. It brings into focus the challenge to an administrator who endeavors to establish a program introducing equality of treatment to female psychiatric patients in today's mental health environment.

Case Study

Step 1—Initiating program plans on the basis of current research findings.

The need to implement a new program at our community hospital was based on knowledge gleaned directly from earlier evaluative research. One of us (M.H.H.) had recently completed a study investigating medical care of mentally ill women that specifically documented the practice of carrying out incomplete physical examinations for female psychiatric inpatients in our hospital (11). Results indicated that the physical examination given upon admission or during a psychiatric stay was often the only maintenance health care received by chronically mentally ill women, and that it was therefore essential that this examination be comprehensive.

However, data from our own hospital revealed a pattern of deferred pelvic examinations that were often not completed before the patient's discharge. Our study concluded that female psychiatric patients were not receiving the kind of generally acceptable physical examination that basic good medical care requires.

After considering these issues and discussing them with colleagues in other hospitals, we decided to correct the situation by instituting routine gynecological examinations for all female psychiatric patients in our hospital. Although we were aware of a fine series of studies carried out by Grunebaum and Abernethy (13, 14, 18–20), in which a program for obstetrical and gynecological care for chronically mentally ill women had been established at a state mental hospital in Massachusetts, there were few other guidelines to help us in establishing the specific gender-related programmatic changes needed for our own general hospital setting. We became aware that we would have to proceed with a certain amount of trial and error.

Step 2—Anticipating and planning for resistances to change.

In our attempts to institute a policy directly responsive to differential gender needs among psychiatric patients, we anticipated the same kinds of resistance that we might face in implementing policies for women in any sector of society, as well as other resistances more particularly related to our own policy-making environment. Specifically, we expected that the administrator would have to be alert to both external, societally influenced stereotypes favoring maintenance of the status quo and other limiting factor and internal priority-setting decisions derived from sources closer to the administrator. Although research had assisted us with the former, in that our study had uncovered many logistical problems common to planning for chronically mentally ill women that we might encounter, the internal limitations were as yet unknown. We decided to deal with the externally derived barriers first.

Step 3—Responding to external barriers: the active phase.

We anticipated that resistance to our plan to provide adequate gynecological care for our chronically mentally ill patients might come from many quarters external to the psychiatric service, because of the complicated process that the plan's implementation would entail. We should need special staff to carry out the examinations, specially equipped treatment rooms, and transportation and chaperone staff, in addition to cooperation from attending psychiatric staff, hospital administration, and the chiefs of the various professional disciplines.

As we prepared to move ahead, we approached all the key people who would be involved, as we might in implementing any new program. Much to our surprise, we were met with enthusiastic support and not with the resistance we had worried about. We found that we were able to form the necessary alliances, because the need for the services we proposed was clear and our goals were simple. The annual report of our chief of psychiatry to the hospital's administration had listed as a goal for fiscal year 1986 to "improve medical/gynecological care for female inpatients, to collaborate with the Chief of Obstetrics and Gynecology to ensure that every female inpatient has a full gynecological examination." Once this policy statement had been made, details and logistics seemed to fall into place readily.

With the enthusiastic support of the chief of obstetrics and gynecology, gynecologists at our hospital offered a protocol and collaborated on the development of a special gynecological consultation form to use in our program. The suggestion was made that our patients be referred for gynecological consultation well into their inpatient stays, once their psychiatric conditions had stabilized or improved somewhat. Patients could then be escorted to the well-equipped offices of the gynecological specialists. For patients unable to be so transported, an appropriate examination would be made available within the psychiatric unit area.

Nursing administrators also supported this plan and encouraged their staff to escort patients to the examining rooms and act as chaperones as needed. Their cooperation in the effort represented a clear response to a compelling need, and the program seemed ready to proceed.

Thus, the external barriers to change that we had anticipated did not in fact limit our progress as we began the implementation process. Since our study had demonstrated a clear state of neglect in patient care, those concerned with implementing the plan were thrilled to be part of redressing the imbalance. Staff members were generally enthusiastic about the notion of improving patient care in this way, and the planning process itself served to reinforce the enthusiasm and to encourage hospital staff to move ahead with a good idea.

Step 4—Weighing conflicting interests: the deliberative phase.

Yet program planning failed to proceed as rapidly as one might expect from the enthusiastic responses throughout the hospital. Surprisingly, it was one of us (M.H.H.), now in an administrative role, who slowed the process down. Internal, rather than external, barriers were intervening to inhibit the innovation process.

The administrator found now that she was faced with having to look at hard questions of priority setting and resource allocation, and the process of change was retarded by the need to weigh conflicting interests. Would the proposed program affect only a small minority of patients and leave others out? Could the extraordinary amount of staff time and resources required justify the program's probable high cost? Could such a program really accomplish its goals? Would it really make a significant enough difference in patient care among chronically mentally ill individuals to justify its implementation?

The administrator was faced with certain paradoxes that intruded at this juncture in the decision-making process. There is, for example, an intrinsic paradox in the notion of equal care. Equality, when based on similarity in procedures and treatments, may not necessarily be equality at all, because high-quality care requires that programs be differentiated so that they may be tailored to individual patients' needs. In terms of physical examination, equality of care for women hardly means "sameness"; rather, it entails differentiated care specific to the particular needs of the subpopulation. However, implementing such differentiated programming might limit the access of other subpopulations to needed care by using up resources.

Thus, the administrator found herself considering two thoughts as she weighed various interests: that providing appropriate physical examinations for women patients, a complicated and costly enterprise, might really be regarded as a special-program need not within the psychiatric services's domain; and that a gynecological examination might not, after all, be such a high priority. Ironically, these were the very arguments that she had anticipated would come from outside sources. Now her decision-making role was complicated: she was experiencing ambivalences about action versus inaction and about progressive versus regressive orientations in patient care.

A second paradox was evident in the fact that subpopulations among the chronically mentally ill (such as women) might simultaneously be overserved and underserved (2, 6). Although women constitute the majority of patients on the inpatient units of our general hospital (during fiscal year 1986 women constituted 61 percent of all admissions), the standard adopted for physical examinations among chronic mental patients responded to the needs of the male patients, who constituted a numerical minority. In the psychiatric service's experience, in short, women had previously been seen as exceptions to the general rule of providing adequate overall physical care.

The administrator's ambivalence was eventually resolved in favor of providing the gynecological examinations. She had reached the conclusion that, in spite of the fact that this potentially costly program would serve only some of the psychiatric service's patients, it was essential for their basic medical care. She was, moreover, supported in this decision by the knowledge that setting up such a program would appropriately combat a common but therapeutically

119

contraindicated tendency to consider chronically mentally ill women as "genderless" (7).

Step 5—Implementing the new program.

In May 1986, a joint memorandum from the administrator and the chief of psychiatry announced the availability of full gynecological examinations for chronic mental patients in the hospital. The following month the chief of psychiatry presented this statement to the psychiatric staff:

> It is Departmental policy to provide a gynecological evaluation for all appropriate female inpatients. The attending psychiatrist should order the examination, which may be performed in the latter part of the hospital stay, perhaps when the patient has privileges and can go to the gynecologist's office. The attending should explain to the patient that we consider a gynecological evaluation an integral part of the comprehensive medical evaluation appropriate for hospitalized psychiatric patients. (Department of Psychiatry staff meeting minutes)

Thus, eight months after the publication of our research demonstrating gender-related inequalities in psychiatric care, a corrective policy was effected. Our work, however, is not done, for we have yet to establish whether this new program will be effective. Comprehensive evaluative research is currently being undertaken toward that end.

Summary and Conclusions

We have now instituted our policy designed to respect gender differences among the chronically mentally ill and specifically to provide for female members of that population equal access to high-quality basic medical care. We are currently in the process of recording evaluative data on the outcomes of this intervention, so that we may assess objectively whether the time and expense are justified. It is possible that our efforts will not uncover the unrecognized gynecological problems that we predicted and that our former research led us to anticipate. On the other hand, we may demonstrate the presence of significant gynecological illness and dysfunction and so be able to alleviate disease and even save lives. In either case our effort

120

has had value in clarifying and documenting the process aspects of implementing innovative programs in the psychiatric inpatient units of general hospitals.

This chapter has examined the administrative process involved in implementing a program to improve the care of chronically mentally ill women in a general hospital psychiatric inpatient unit by providing them with full gynecological examinations in the hospital. In our case study we have shown that research demonstrating need may actually be translated into action; it may be used to mobilize support for a program that seeks to redress imbalances.

However, research results alone do not determine the direction or the speed of program planning and program implementation, no matter how clear and justified the goals of the new intervention might be. Administrative constraints are also significant forces affecting program design and development. Programmatic decisions must be weighed in the light of the costs and benefits involved. Because our particular program called for services to be provided exclusively to female patients, it touched on issues that generally do not arise when chronically mentally ill are regarded as genderless individuals.

In this instance, we were able to rationalize implementing the new program on the grounds that it would benefit a majority of the chronically mentally ill patients enrolled in our hospital, that it constituted good public health care, and that it had the clear support of staff in both the psychiatric service and the gynecological service. By reviewing facts, examining paradoxes, and seeking to adhere to the highest standards of patient care, the administrator was ultimately able to proceed by implementing a program that seeks to fulfill the mandates for continuity of care and individual regard for the needs of all patients.

References

1. Bachrach LL: Continuity of care for chronic mental patients: a conceptual analysis. Am J Psychiatry 138:1449–1456, 1981
2. Bachrach LL: Planning services for chronically mentally ill patients. Bull Menninger Clin 47:163–188, 1983
3. Granet R, Talbott JA: The continuity agent: creating a new role to bridge the gaps in the mental health system. Hosp Community Psychiatry 29:132–133, 1978

4. Stroul B: Models of Community Support Services: Approaches to Helping Persons with Long Term Mental Illness. Rockville, MD, Community Support Program, National Institute of Mental Health, 1986

5. Bachrach LL: Deinstitutionalization and women: assessing the consequences of public policy. Am Psychol 39:1171–1177, 1984

6. Carmon E, Russo N, Miller J: Inequality and women's mental health: an overview. Am J Psychiatry 138:1319–1330, 1981

7. Test M, Berlin S: Issues of special concern to chronically mentally ill women. Professional Psychology 12:136–145, 1981

8. Lewine R: Sex differences in age of symptom onset and first hospitalization in schizophrenia. Am J Orthopsychiatry 50:326–322, 1980

9. Seeman M: Gender differences in schizophrenia. Can J Psychiatry 27:107–112, 1982

10. Bardenstein K, McGlashan T: Gender differences in schizophrenia. Presented at the annual meeting of the American Psychiatric Association, Washington, DC, 15 May 1986

11. Handel M: Deferred pelvic examinations: a purposeful omission in the care of mentally ill women. Hosp Community Psychiatry 36:1070–1073, 1985

12. Seeman M: Schizophrenic men and women require different treatment programs. Journal of Psychiatric Treatment and Evaluation 5:143–148, 1983

13. Grunebaum H, Abernethy V: The family planning attitudes, practices and motivation of mental patients. Am J Psychiatry 128:96–110, 1971

14. Abernethy V, Grunebaum H: Toward a family planning program in psychiatric hospitals. Am J Public Health 62:1638–1642, 1971

15. Greenblatt M, Sharaf M, Stone E: Dynamics of Institutional Change: The Hospital in Transition. Pittsburgh, University of Pittsburgh Press, 1971

16. Barton W: What's new in administration. Hosp Community Psychiatry 24:441–443, 1983

17. Arce A, Adams M, Woods J, et al: Cost containment in a community mental health center. Hosp Community Psychiatry 31:103–107, 1980

18. Grunebaum H, Abernethy V, Clough L, et al: Staff attitudes toward a family planning service in the mental hospital. Community Ment Health J 11:280–285, 1975
19. Grunebaum H, Abernethy V: Ethical issues in family planning for hospitalized psychiatric patients. Am J Psychiatry 132:236–240, 1975
20. Abernethy V, Grunebaum H: Family planning in two psychiatric hospitals: a preliminary report. Fam Plann Perspect 5:94–99, 1973

Chapter 9

Homelessness Among Chronically Mentally Ill Women

MARSHA A. MARTIN, D.S.W.

Chapter 9

Homelessness Among Chronically Mentally Ill Women

Women and children form a substantial subset of the homeless. They have specific needs for program planning, such as safety, medical care, food, clothing, shelter, personal hygiene, and financial support. Many in this population suffer from serious mental illness, and treatment resources must include access to medical care. The author of this chapter delineates the scope of the problem and describes a specific New York City program.

Chronically mentally ill women are individuals who have varying problems and needs. Some are women who have been formally diagnosed with chronic psychotic disorders and treated with a variety of therapeutic interventions. Some have been discharged from state mental hospitals to the care of family members and have made successful linkages to community resources and support systems. Others are women who have been released to the community for care, sometimes to a single-room-occupancy (SRO) hotel or a board-and-care home, with or without a medication regimen, and often only with a hope that both the community and the patient might adapt to one another.

Still others are women who have never been institutionalized in a state mental hospital because of the impact of deinstitutionalization on current hospital admission policies. Commonly referred to as members of the "young adult chronically mentally ill" patient population, which is today emerging as a service group with special needs, these women are typically impaired to a degree where they are socially inadequate. They tend to exhibit extensive symptomatology as well as a need for structure; and they represent a challenge to traditional mental health services, which seem unable to reach them.

This chapter describes a special subgroup of chronically mentally ill women who have become homeless, and discusses the problems that service providers encounter in their attempts to serve these individuals. Several case histories are provided, and effective program strategies, including a stepwise treatment plan, are discussed.

Defining Homelessness

Homelessness, as defined in the *International Encyclopedia of the Social Sciences*, is a condition of detachment from society. It is characterized by the absence or attenuation of the affiliative bonds that link settled persons to a network of interconnected social structures. Homelessness may take many forms, depending on the type of detachment and on local circumstances. Homeless families and homeless men, so far as can be determined, are found in all large societies. Homeless women and children, by contrast, are relatively more rare. Their appearance generally denotes widespread societal disorder and instability (1).

In the United States today, the estimated number of homeless men, women, and children combined ranges from 350,000 to more than 2.5 million persons nationwide (2, 3). In some cities—for example, Los Angeles, Chicago, Houston, and New York—the number of homeless individuals is estimated to be anywhere from 25,000 to more than 70,000 persons. The "guesstimated" percentage of mentally ill persons among the homeless ranges from 30 percent to more than 90 percent of the total, depending on such factors as the geographical location of the population; whether the population is found inside or outside a service facility such as a shelter; the philosophy and area of specialization of the facility; and the diagnostic assessment process, including what specific instrument is used to identify psychopathology (4–6).

Irrespective of the specific percentage of the homeless population estimated as being mentally ill, members of this population are defined by the fact that they suffer from chronic conditions that are, according to a dictionary definition, marked by long duration, by frequent recurrence over a long time, and often by "slowly progressing seriousness." Their diagnoses include schizophrenia, manic-depressive disease, alcoholism (even in recovery), organic brain syndrome associated with senility or syphilis, mental retardation, and certain drug addictions and personality disorders (7).

Some vignettes illustrate the varied characteristics of female members of the homeless mentally ill population:

> With no fear to protect her, Florence cannot be let out alone. At 30, she has spent most of her life in an institution. She is not disturbed, just slow. When she feels well, she speaks clearly and can read. Most of the time, her speech is slurred. She gets a welfare check but when she has money she drinks, and then wanders off to sleep in the park. She has been attacked, beaten and robbed. (8)

> She was called the cellophane lady because of the way she wrapped her legs and feet to protect them from the Philadelphia cold. It didn't work: last winter Lillian Roseborogh nearly lost her limbs because of hypothermia. Even so, the 65-year-old woman refused to be removed from the street where she lives—just a block from her daughter's apartment. She insisted that she was ruled by the spirit of the "jing-jing" and that if she went inside before the government provided shelter for all street people, she would die. (9)

> Rosa is a survivor. At 55, she has lived on Los Angeles' skid row for more than 20 years and slept in cheap hotels until none would have her. Rosa has delusions. She imagines that her sons, taken from her years ago, are in danger. She can be hard to handle then. Barred from hotels, Rosa moved into the area's parking lots. (9)

> Fantasy and reality merge in Emily's world. She rattles on endlessly, with elaborate plans to feed and house the homeless. "I'm one of the most allergic persons in the U.S.," she says. "Put me in jail and I can't last more than fifty hours, even in the very nice jails they have here. I couldn't take the food. I eat three pounds of vegetables a day." But she sometimes scrounges scraps from a fast food outlet. "Recycling," she calls it. Medication makes her ill. "I gain fifty pounds every time I'm in the hospital." For more than a year she has slept in an abandoned building with no electricity. (8)

Program Description

From the spring of 1981 until the fall of 1985, I directed the Midtown Outreach Program of the Manhattan Bowery Corporation, a mobile mental health outreach program staffed with psychiatrists, masters'-level social workers and nurse-practitioners, licensed practical nurses, and mental health aides. The program was designed specifically to draw into treatment homeless mentally ill individuals in the greater Times Square area of New York City. The women served by the program are very similar to those described in the case vignettes from the literature that I have just cited.

In its early phases, the program offered information, referral, and escort to service agencies where homeless women's basic needs —food, clothing, shelter, showers, and so forth—could be met. Included among the agencies served by the outreach program were a number of public and private shelters, drop-in centers, soup kitchens, and showering and delousing facilities. The street outreach teams, consisting of trained social workers, provided outreach services to homeless individuals between the hours of 9 a.m. and 11 p.m., Monday through Friday.

During the initial 12 to 18 months of the program's operation, outreach workers also responded to the concrete needs of those persons who they approached on the streets and in transportation facilities. They made assessments of these individuals to determine which of them were in need of medical and psychiatric interventions—a process that sometimes resulted in either voluntary or involuntary escort to a municipal hospital emergency room. Such hospital escorts would often end in seven- to ten-hour waits in the emergency room, while decisions regarding possible admission were being made.

In approaching homeless mentally ill individuals, outreach workers began by concentrating on persons' articulated and perceived needs: They started with "where the homeless person was": undomiciled, hungry, lousy, and disheveled in appearance. However, it was clear to these workers that many of the individuals approached by them also required medical and psychiatric care.

The need for homeless mentally ill individuals to have access to medical and psychiatric services became even more apparent as outreach teams improved their assessment and diagnostic skills. Workers were discovering a relationship between the level of functioning as evidenced by utilization of available services and the level of psychiatric and medical impairment. In addition, many of the individuals approached by the outreach teams showed not only clear behavioral signs of such chronic mental illnesses as schizophrenia, depression, and organic brain syndrome, but also evidence of such chronic physical illnesses as diabetes, congestive heart failure, upper and lower respiratory infections, hypertension, obesity, and a variety of dermatological problems. Often these physical conditions resulted in individuals' inability to utilize fully what services were available to them. Women represented between 45 and 55 percent of the monthly and annual caseloads.

Addition of Medical and Psychiatric Services

The initial program to provide street outreach services to the homeless in midtown Manhattan has now been expanded by the addition of a medical-psychiatric component to the program. Medical-psychiatric teams now offer on-site services from 9 a.m. until 9 p.m., Monday through Friday, in seven selected shelters and drop-in centers. They also provide much needed medical and psychiatric backup to the street outreach component.

The medical-psychiatric component offers an array of medical and psychiatric services to homeless mentally ill individuals. Included are mental status evaluations, diagnostic workups, physical assessments, prescription and administration of medications, follow-up care, disability documentation, patient care education groups, and staff consultation in regularly scheduled clinic visits to the specified service sites. Four of the seven shelters included in the program serve homeless women exclusively, two serve both men and women, and one serves men only.

In contrast to the population of individuals approached on the streets, where women and men are roughly equally represented, the population served in the facility component of the outreach program shows a preponderance of women. Women currently account for 73 percent of all cases. Fifty-two percent of all cases, men and women combined, are over 40 years of age; and 45 percent are white, 45 percent black, and 10 percent Hispanic or Asian-American. For both sexes combined, 47 percent are diagnosed with schizophrenia; among women only, the comparable figure is 53 percent. Many of the women are on neuroleptics prescribed and monitored by the medical-psychiatric treatment teams.

Treating Homeless Mentally Ill Women

The approach used by the medical-psychiatric team to treat chronically mentally ill homeless women has evolved through actual experience in working with the target population. Drop-in center and shelter guests become patients of the medical-psychiatric team in one of three ways: self-referral, referral by facility staff, or identification by street outreach staff.

Initial screening and intake assessments are conducted by the mental health aide and the licensed practical nurse. The nurse-practitioner or physician's assistant and the psychiatrist then see the woman for further evaluation after the initial intake procedures have been completed. A team discussion follows, and a treatment plan is set into action.

The team carries with it all supplies, medications, and equipment necessary for facilitating immediate treatments and interventions. In addition, the team may order laboratory tests and complete electrocardiograms without having to refer the patient to a hospital. Assessment and treatment protocols that correspond to common complaints and illnesses within the population have now been developed.

Many of the women seen by the medical-psychiatric treatment team have a history of running away from hospitals or residential facilities and of noncompliance with medications and aftercare recommendations. As a result, they have often been labeled "hard to reach," "hard to work with," and "hard to rehabilitate." By establishing a therapeutic alliance with each patient at the shelter or drop-in center and by providing medications and follow-up without making it necessary for the patient to undergo protracted intake and the stressfulness of waiting in line, the team is able to respond more readily than in the past to homeless women's special needs. Through this approach the team has been able to prevent acute decompensations, reduce demands on emergency rooms, and otherwise prevent unnecessary hospitalizations.

The medical-psychiatric outreach program was designed to engage the homeless mentally ill in treatment and to provide basic survival services and medical and psychiatric care until such time as the individual patient can be referred to an agency in the community. If a patient can maintain a minimal level of functioning and remain stable in the loosely structured shelter/drop-in center environment, she is considered to be a better eventual candidate for care in the traditional psychiatric service system.

The program thus responds to two kinds of concerns in reaching homeless mentally ill women. First, it aids shelter and drop-in center staff in assisting those guests who are chronically mentally ill; and, second, it assists traditional mental health service providers who are searching for effective methods for connecting, or re-connecting, with those members of their patient population who have become homeless.

Program Interventions

The specific manner in which the medical-psychiatric team executes its functions and responsibilities is illustrated in the following case examples. Names of the patients have been altered to protect their identities.

Mary Jones, a middle-aged white woman diagnosed with para-noid schizophrenia, has been living off and on the street for between two and four years. She has a history of several psychiatric hospital-izations characterized by bizarre delusions: people who are putting parts of animals into her body and spirits that are controlling her mind. She has been removed from the street by police on several occasions, hospitalized in a municipal hospital, and rereleased to the street. On several occasions the team has been able to assist her in finding shelter and, at least once, found an SRO room for her. However, she eventually lost that room as the result of her poor hygiene, her habit of rummaging through garbage receptacles in the hotel lobby, and her letting the shower overrun to cause numerous floods. Refusing to accept any further help, she returned to the street.

Ms. Jones was approached on several occasions on the street corner where she had set up "house." She had specific areas for sleeping, washing up, bathing, eating, and so forth. Eventually, she became somewhat more receptive to the team members, so that they were able to evaluate her further. She remained suspicious and disturbed and continued to have bizarre paranoid and somatic delu-sions: People were eating her brain, spiders were coming out of her body, and the like. Her legs and hands were swollen, and there was the possibility of a vaginal infection. She was hospitalized involun-tarily at a municipal hospital and later transferred to a state psychi-atric facility, where she remains.

In some instances, the medical-psychiatric treatment team's in-terventions may be undermined, because of difficulties in maintain-ing patients in inpatient care. Kathryn Appleby, a black woman in

133

her late 40s, is a chronic paranoid schizophrenic with a ten-year history of hospitalizations in state psychiatric institutions. She came to the drop-in center and requested help against people trying to kill her. She was started on a small dose of fluphenazine decanoate every week. Eventually, the dose was increased to 50 mg intramuscularly every other week. Because of a history of alcoholism and occasional alcoholic binges, she also started receiving thiamine 100 mg once a day. Her condition was somewhat stabilized for an eight-week period, but she had to be hospitalized because of the high risk of suicide. However, she left the hospital on her own after 72 hours without appropriate discharge planning.

Sometimes, on the other hand, the medical-psychiatric outreach team's interventions prove to be quite effective in helping patients to avoid unneeded hospitalizations. Jim and Barbara Whitehead are a married couple served by the team. Jim is a middle-aged white male with mild dementia. He was started on a low dose of haloperidol. Shortly after the medical-psychiatric team began to work with him, he was hospitalized when he began to smear feces on the walls of the shelter and to attack boys on the street sexually. He remained in the municipal hospital until he was transferred to a nursing home. Barbara, a middle-aged black woman, began showing signs of exacerbation of chronic paranoid delusions and marked agitation after she learned that Jim would have to go to a nursing home. She accepted voluntary hospitalization and is back at the shelter on perphenazine. She is compliant with the medication, much calmer, cooperative with the shelter staff and the outreach team, and is no longer acutely disturbed by her "prison control system."

The team also provides some case management functions. However, given the nature of the patient population, success in such efforts is variable and sometimes unpredictable. Sandy Carter, a black woman in her mid-twenties, was brought to the shelter by a street outreach team after several approaches to her in the train station. After a few nights in the shelter, Sandy began to talk to herself and became agitated to the point of disrupting the shelter environment. It was explained to her that she would be permitted to stay in the shelter only if she would agree to see the doctor. She left the shelter but eventually returned more disorganized and more disoriented than before; she was also suffering from auditory hallucinations.

134

Ms. Carter was eventually stabilized on medication, and housing was made available to her at a nearby SRO hotel. She continued to visit the shelter on a daily basis for her medications and her meals. She finally decided to return to her mother's house in another state. Efforts were made to enroll her in a mental health clinic at her destination, but she left before final arrangements could be made.

These illustrations not only demonstrate the activities of the medical-psychiatric outreach program but they also underscore the difficulties inherent in meeting the treatment needs of chronically mentally ill individuals who live on the streets. Furthermore, they point up some very important issues relating to homelessness. Martin Begun (11) writes that "probably no one, however sane, could remain physically and emotionally intact after even a week in these conditions." For chronically mentally ill women, the street, homelessness, and the shelter experience itself complicate the rehabilitative process that is part of effective psychiatric care; they make the road to indoor living an extremely difficult one to negotiate. The condition of homelessness is a devastating reality. Without a home, a woman has no place in which to base her identity, no stability, no foundation. And society still strongly suggests that "a woman's place is in the home."

Yet "home" has become a truly unattainable goal for many chronically mentally ill homeless women. An examination of these women's survival needs, and of the strategies they develop to deal with their circumstances, may help us to understand some of the reasons that implementing change is so difficult.

Treatment Planning and Survival Strategies

It has been demonstrated that, generally speaking, chronically mentally ill women do not make an eccentric or idiosyncratic choice to be homeless; rather, they become or remain homeless in order to survive. Thus, living on the street most often represents a survival technique for these women, not just a temporary solution to a situational problem (12). A "survival drive" that characterizes these women sparks a process of adaptation that continues so long as they remain homeless. Basic survival strategies include the creation of personalized methods for acquiring such necessities as food, clothing, showers, shelter, and financial support. When these kinds of services are not offered to them institutionally, homeless mentally ill women may be remarkably creative in finding their own personalized alternatives.

In addition to these survival strategies, homeless mentally ill women also evolve certain maintenance strategies to lessen the immediate impact of stress and to enable them to maintain some sense of self-worth. These strategies include such defense mechanisms as denial ("I don't live on the street"), rationalization ("I like being outdoors"), and fantasy play and self-entertainment (singing, dancing, chatting with passersby, teasing children, and so forth). By means of these strategies homeless mentally ill women are able to remove themselves from the everyday stresses associated with living on the streets (12).

In many cases chronically mentally ill women become and remain homeless in part because they find the random care offered them on the streets preferable to that which they might receive in other environments, familial or institutional. Passersby may inquire about their health, give them food, money, and clothing, and generally look out for them. These kinds of events result in a kind of intermittent reinforcement that traditional service providers may find difficult to extinguish when they offer alternatives to life on the street (12). Yet treatment planners must take this kind of information into consideration if they are to provide appropriate services. It is not enough to offer the homeless mentally ill woman shelter and a hot meal, for these commodities, essential as they are, are not enough. They must be supplemented by rehabilitative efforts that acknowledge the adaptive process, as well as the special strengths and abilities that individual women often possess.

Thus, treatment interventions not only must offer external alternatives to living on the streets, but also must contribute to the restructuring of these women's ego realities. Stated differently, programs for homeless mentally ill women must seek to teach the "rules" of indoor living to homeless women sympathetically and respectfully (13). They must strive to offer to these women autonomy and anonymity when sought. In addition, they must respond to the multiple needs of homeless mentally ill women without overriding the life choices they have made based on their own sense of survival. And they must, at least initially, utilize program eligibility criteria that do not contravene these women's current lifestyles.

Phases of Treatment

As the result of its intensive work with homeless mentally ill women, the Midtown Outreach Program has developed a stepwise treatment approach that has general applicability in programs targeted toward homeless women: It may be used effectively by shelter staffs, medical and psychiatric personnel, and various social service professionals who seek to serve homeless mentally ill women and engage them in care. It is an approach that provides the basis for an effective therapeutic relationship and for identification of the woman's special strengths so that they may be used in restructuring ego-reality.

As in every therapeutic process, treatment must begin where the patient is: mentally ill and homeless. The first phase of treatment is devoted to addressing the woman's concrete needs. Often, even when a homeless mentally ill woman rejects more extensive interventions, she may tolerate assistance that responds to her basic needs. Small shelters and drop-in centers may be very important resources during the initial phases of working with these individuals, as they offer basic services that address immediate needs.

The presence of an outreach mental health team to provide backup clinical support is also important during this initial period. Basic questions must be answered at this time: How is the woman meeting her basic needs? What does she do for food, clothing, shelter, personal hygiene, socialization, safety, and financial support? How does she handle these needs? Does she have a system in place to meet immediate requirements? Are her strategies adaptive or maladaptive? Is she successful? Asking such questions is important to identify situations in which the woman's behavior is organized, integrated, and basically appropriate. Answers may supply clues about the woman's level of functioning to service providers who are looking for strengths to tap as they urge her to accept traditional mental health services—that is, strengths that may prove to be critical in providing a foundation for indoor living.

After stabilization occurs, more extensive psychiatric and medical interventions are usually possible. However, this period of treatment is, at best, unpredictable. Homeless mentally ill women, often afraid of social contact, may get close and then flee out of disappointment or fear of rejection. There will probably be repetitions of such behavior before any notable improvement occurs. Thus, this second phase of care may prove to be unrewarding and frustrating to service providers unless they learn to accept very small goals, such as the woman's showering once a week, or her eating lunch at a soup kitchen, or her remembering to take medications at least once a week, as evidence of her progress.

The second or middle phase of treatment with homeless mentally ill women is directed at sustaining the therapeutic relationship through identifying the individual's current skills and helping her to develop new ones. This is the period of encouragement. For example, because many homeless mentally ill women are eligible for disability benefits, it might be well to encourage them to apply for those benefits at this time, perhaps with the assistance of an advocate.

Once the homeless woman has begun to respond to offers of assistance in meeting her basic needs on an ongoing basis and once she is likely to continue taking medications, it is important that she be provided with assurances that services and resources will be available to her continually, as she needs them. It is also very important that the service provider maintain an attitude of acceptance of the woman's life circumstances during this second phase. Therapists must be especially tuned in to the woman's feelings during this period. If a homeless woman becomes too anxious, it is better to postpone involvement with community services until she expresses feelings of security.

It must be acknowledged that this second phase may well be a time that may be terrifying for the homeless mentally ill woman. Involvement with community services beyond those that meet her basic needs requires her to participate actively in her own care—an expectation that may frighten her. Some women disappear during this phase. Others, however, show eagerness to pursue rehabilitative goals.

During these first two phases, the focus is on addressing the homeless mentally ill woman's basic needs and beginning work on reestablishing her connections with the community. In the third and final phase of work the focus must be on supporting the woman's attempts at indoor living. For many homeless women, moving "back indoors," much as they may want to do so, is a task requiring a tremendous amount of encouragement. These women often have lived on the streets for some time and have had no responsibility for keeping a household of any size intact.

This is also a step that may result in the termination of the therapeutic relationship. The process may evoke powerful feelings in the homeless mentally ill woman: a sense of loss, anger, and potential abandonment. At the same time, the woman may have some feelings of success and mastery. It is these latter feelings that will allow her to move forward and that may lead her to an improved sense of self by elevating her self-esteem.

The most important aspect of this final phase in treating homeless mentally ill women is to help each individual to maintain the gains she has already made, to master the separation, and to utilize the services and the resources that the community has to offer to her.

Providing care to homeless mentally ill women is a difficult but not always insurmountable task. It requires patience, dedication, and, above all, respect for the woman's self and her right to a comfortable existence.

References

1. Caplow T, Bahr HR, Sternberg D, et al: Homelessness, in International Encyclopedia of the Social Sciences. New York, Macmillan, 1968, pp 494–498
2. Hombs ME, Snyder M: Homeless in America: A Forced March to Nowhere. Washington, DC, Community for Creative Nonviolence, 1982
3. United States Department of Housing and Urban Development: A Report to the Secretary on the Homeless and Emergency Shelters. Washington, DC, United States Department of Housing and Urban Development, 1984
4. Bassuk E: The homeless problem. Sci Am 241:40–45, 1984
5. Hoffman S: Who Are the Homeless? A Study of Randomly Selected Men Who Use the New York City Shelters. Albany, NY, State Office of Mental Health, May 1982
6. Roth D, Bean J, Lust N, et al: Homelessness in Ohio: A Study of People in Need. Columbus, Ohio Department of Mental Health, 1985.
7. Minkoff K: A map of the chronic mental patient, in The Chronic Mental Patient. Edited by Talbott JA. Washington, DC, American Psychiatric Association, 1978, pp 11–37

8. Mothner I: Out on the streets. GEO 4:78–91, 1983
9. Alter J, Stille A, Doherty F, et al: Homeless in America. Newsweek, 2 January 1984, pp 20–29
10. Manhattan Bowery Corporation Case Records. New York, 1985
11. Begun M: The mentally ill homeless need more than shelter. New York University Physician 41:67–70, 1985
12. Martin MA: Strategies of Adaptation: Coping Patterns of the Urban Transient Female. D.S.W. dissertation, New York, Columbia University, 1982
13. Martin MA: Shaping Behavior and Re-Structuring Ego Reality. Presented at the Hunter College School of Social Work Clinical Conference, 16 May 1985

Chapter 10

The Iatrogenic Creation of Psychiatric Chronicity in Women

JEFFREY L. GELLER, M.D., M.P.H.
MARK R. MUNETZ, M.D.

Chapter 10

The Iatrogenic Creation of Psychiatric Chronicity in Women

Without belaboring the point, we must emphasize again the need for historical understanding and perspective if we are to face the problems of the future. This chapter describes the experiences of female patients in the past and looks at some current gender-specific issues, especially the use of neuroleptics.

*T*he history of American institutional psychiatry is rich with published reports by former patients who have railed against the injudicious and ill-conceived nature of their psychiatric confinement. In 1833, Robert Fuller wrote:

> Where one has been falsely accused, imprisoned and persecuted nearly unto death, it is both his right and duty to make such an exposition of the whole affair as will tend to prevent its recurrence . . . The McLean Asylum for the Insane possesses a large share of popular favour . . . To the passing stranger, it excites no other emotions than those of beauty, comfort, benevolence and joy . . . But let him go with me within its world: let him hear the groans of the distressed: let him see its inmates shut up with bars and bolts: let him see how deserted . . . neglected and cruelly treated . . . and his views of that institution will change. (1)

Nine years later, Elizabeth Stone echoed these concerns:

> Feeling that the public is very much deceived concerning the treatment and situation of a poor afflicted class of the human family, who are placed in the McLean Asylum . . . I will expose this matter to the public, in behalf of the afflicted, in connection with the *awful, brutal outrage* [emphasis in original] that has been committed upon me. . . . (2)

Such accounts can readily be found in writings of the second half of the nineteenth century. The most vocal and prolific campaigner against the injustices of institutionalization was Elizabeth Parsons Ware Packard, who indicated that "Insane asylums are the *'Inquisitions'* of the American government" (3). Adeline Lunt wrote in 1871:

But the modern system of treatment of the insane proves that, shut within a building a man may be more completely cut off from all that pertains to this world and its interests, than he could be at the remotest ends of the earth, or beyond all reach of civilization. (4)

Throughout the twentieth century, former patients have continued to make public their concerns about psychiatric institutions and psychiatric treatment. In 1902, Kate Lee indicated,

Whatever treatment is given at the asylum seems to consist of regular hours, long nights of sleep, low diet, a daily walk and discipline.... The term hospital, which is frequently used for the asylum, should be changed ... and the term "patient" so often used there, is evidently misleading, as the inmates are not patients in any true sense of the word. (5)

In 1947, Laura Jefferson wrote,

The State has adjudged me insane and I am no longer responsible for anything, so it is stupid and senseless for me to try and salvage anything out of the tangle. But, since the tangle is I, I cannot let it lay as it is.... I still have a life on my hands—even though it must be lived out in an insane asylum. Though I have lost every encounter, I am still not dismissed from the conflict. (6)

And in 1985, an anonymous woman protested,

I just want to say that I'm proud to be a madwoman, and that I couldn't have survived any other way. Although I've been tortured with 17 shock treatments, with Prolixin, with Lithium, with being mind-fucked in this society, at least I know my mind.... I'm not going to live out my life passively. I don't want the straightjacket. I've already been institutionalized and I'm not going to wear it on the outside. (7)

144

Statement of Problem

It is undoubtedly true that the vast majority of former psychiatric inpatients lack a combination of the wherewithal, the means, and the motivation to publicize the details of their patienthood even when they have had serious questions about the legitimacy of that former status. But there are tens of thousands of individuals who spent prolonged periods in America's state hospitals before the era of deinstitutionalization, who now live in the community. Some of these former state hospital residents are seen in outpatient psychiatric treatment, but they remain quiet on the subject of their institutional stays. Usually they are not asked, and their old records are rarely reviewed.

Our interest in one subset of this population was piqued during the course of our work in a mental health setting serving predominantly schizophrenic outpatients. We noted a group of patients who had either no psychosis or had had a short psychotic episode, followed by prolonged inpatient treatment and years of prescribed neuroleptic medications. These latter patients, after having been discharged from that hospitalization, functioned at a reasonably high level, with few decompensations. We also noted that the outpatients who fit this pattern were, by and large, women.

To get a sense of who these people are, consider the following case vignette.

Case Study

Ms. M is a 62-year-old, white, divorced woman who has historically carried the diagnosis of chronic undifferentiated schizophrenia. She had a high level of functioning during young adulthood, evidenced by graduation from high school with a B average, completion of a beautician training program, an active social life, eight years of full-time employment, and four years of marriage before the onset of her psychiatric illness at age 27. Her initial symptom complex included overwhelming feelings of sadness, sleep disturbances, withdrawal from interpersonal relationships, decreased performance at work, and marital discord. Ms. M's symptoms progressed to paranoid delusions, agitation, assaultiveness, and homicidal ideas toward her husband. After attempting to stab her husband, she was admitted to a state hospital.

Ms. M's psychotic symptoms cleared within four months. She began to work in the hospital beauty shop. Within a year, Ms. M was working full time as a beautician at the state hospital. Ms. M's husband divorced her after she had been in the state hospital three years.

In the mid-1950s, Ms. M was started on chlorpromazine despite the fact that she had been free of psychotic symptoms for at least five years. During the next ten years Ms. M remained in the state hospital, worked in the beauty shop, and was treated with 500 mg of chlorpromazine per day.

In 1966, Ms. M was discharged but told that she would need to stay on medication for the rest of her life if she wanted to avoid returning to the state hospital. Within six months of discharge, Ms. M had a full-time job as a nurse's aide. Two years after discharge, Ms. M's medication was changed from chlorpromazine to trifluoperazine. Ms. M recalls again being told how important it was that she faithfully take her medications to avoid becoming psychotic and remembers how frightened she was that this might occur. In 1976, at the insistence of clinical staff, systematic gradual decreases were made in Ms. M's medication. Ms. M was worried about these decreases and repeatedly expressed the fear she would become psychotic again. In 1980, note was made that Ms. M had moderate tardive dyskinesia. At this point she had been out of the hospital for 14 years, working full time, living independently, and maintaining good social relationships with neighbors and family. There had been no indication of any exacerbation of symptoms even during periods of stress. Recommendations were made to Ms. M that she consider further tapering of medication with the goal of total discontinuation, in view of her good functioning and her tardive dyskinesia. Ms. M refused, expressing the fear she would become ill and stating she knew she needed the medication to "stay well." She has not altered her position in the ensuing six years.

In this paper we report on our initial investigation of this patient population and focus on the following questions: What patients are in this group, and are they in fact predominantly women? If they are, how do we account for this pattern of care and treatment and its differential application to women? What has been the morbidity resulting from how these individuals were and continue to be treated? Finally, what are the implications of what we have found for future psychiatric care and treatment?

Method

The study was conducted at the Cognitive Disorders Clinic (CDC) of the Western Psychiatric Institute and Clinic (WPIC). The CDC is the outpatient division of the schizophrenia module. It functions as a public-sector clinic for an urban catchment area. The demographics of the CDC patient population at the time of the study are presented in Table 1.

CDC staff with case loads (three psychiatrists, four psychiatric nurse-clinicians, a social worker, and a bachelor's-level nurse clinician) were asked to identify all patients who had had brief (or nonexistent) psychotic episodes, followed by a long hospitalization

TABLE 1. Demographics of Cognitive Disorders Clinic Population

Characteristic	No.	(%)
Sex		
Male	185	(46)
Female	217	(54)
Race		
Caucasian	276	(69)
Black	121	(30)
Other	5	(1)
Marital status		
Never married	244	(61)
Married	49	(12)
Separated	25	(6)
Divorced	55	(14)
Widowed	29	(7)
Employment		
Full-time	40	(10)
Part-time	32	(8)
Homemaker	54	(13)
Unemployed	255	(63)
Retired	6	(1)
Student	12	(3)
Unknown	3	(1)
Age		
<35	147	(37)
35–55	158	(40)
>55	97	(23)
Age by sex		
<35	M: 91	(62)
	F: 56	(38)
35–55	M: 77	(49)
	F: 81	(51)
>55	M: 17	(18)
	F: 80	(82)

(measurable in months to years), and at least several years of neuroleptic treatment. Criteria were intentionally left vague, and clinicians were asked to err on the side of being overinclusive. By this method 47 patients were identified, 39 women and 8 men.

The authors examined these 47 cases by reviewing the WPIC institutional records. In those instances where the WPIC record did not contain copies of the state hospital record, signed releases were obtained from patients, and the records were procured from the state hospital. We applied the following inclusion criteria: an index hospitalization characterized by psychosis of less than six months and an inpatient stay of greater than one year; the index hospitalization could not have been preceded by more than two prior psychiatric admissions; at least five years of treatment with neuroleptic medication; and a history following the index hospitalization that was not characterized by repeated psychiatric admissions. The authors reached consensus on including or excluding each of the 47 cases.

Results

Twenty-three patients met the inclusion criteria. Of these, 22 were women; 1 was a man. This gender distribution is significantly different from that of the clinic population $\chi^2 = 15.61$, $df = 1$, $p < 0.001$). The remainder of the discussion of the results focuses on the 22 women.

The demographic characteristics of the 22 women and 1 man are defined in Table 2. There were 20 caucasians and 3 blacks, with a mean current age of 63.4 years old (range, 43–76 years). Twelve women had no admissions before the index admission, five had one admission, and five had two admissions. The mean age at first psychiatric admission was 32.6 years (range, 18–47 years); at index hospitalization it was 36.2 years (range, 18–50 years). At the index admission, six women were married, three separated, four divorced, one widowed, and eight were never married.

A description of the index hospitalization for the 23 patients is presented in Table 3. The mean length of hospitalization was 141 months (range, 13–528 months). All but one woman were diagnosed as schizophrenic. Twenty-one of the women received neuroleptic medication during this admission. In addition, 6 received antidepressant medication and 10 received some form of shock therapy.

148

TABLE 2. Demographic Characteristics of Patients Meeting Inclusion Criteria

Case	Sex	Age	Race[a]	No. of Hospitalizations Before Index Admission	Age at First Admission	Marital Status at Index Admission	Age at Index Admission
1	F	66	C	None	47	Married	47
2	F	71	C	2	23	Divorced	31
3	F	71	B	1	46	Separated	47
4	F	44	C	None	30	Married	30
5	F	73	C	2	38	Married	50
6	F	76	C	1	37	Divorced	49
7	F	58	C	None	32	Married	32
8	F	61	C	None	38	Single	38
9	F	69	C	1	37	Separated	41
10	F	51	B	1	27	Separated	31
11	F	43	B	None	20	Married	20
12	F	63	C	None	33	Single	33
13	F	58	C	None	35	Single	35
14	F	68	C	None	22	Single	22
15	F	71	C	None	19	Single	19
16	F	69	C	2	33	Single	36
17	F	62	C	None	47	Single	47
18	F	72	C	None	41	Widowed	41
19	F	65	C	1	28	Divorced	34
20	F	67	C	2	18	Single	45
21	F	59	C	None	35	Divorced	35
22	F	57	C	2	32	Married	34
23	M	53	C	None	33	Single	33

[a]C, Caucasian; B, black.

TABLE 3. Hospitalization Index Circumstances

Case	Length of Hospital Stay (mos.)	Length of Psychotic Symptoms (mos.)	Length of Diagnosis	Time of Neuroleptics	Antidepressants and/or ECT	Off-Ward Job	Changes in Social Circumstances During Hospitalization
1	40	1.5	Schizophrenia, paranoid	Chlorpromazine	No	Hospital cashier through most of hospitalization	End of marriage
2	399	2	Schizophrenia, residual	Thioridazine	Antidepressants, ECT	Cafeteria worker; "succeeded at almost anything she tried to do"	Lost contact with all siblings
3	82	1	Acute brain syndrome, 2° alcohol, and Schizophrenia, chronic undifferentiated	Chlorpromazine, then trifluoperazine	No		
4	16	3	Schizophrenia, acute	Trifluoperazine	No		Divorced; lost contact with son
5	54	2	Schizophrenia, paranoid	Chlorpromazine, then fluphenazine	No	Multiple jobs; labeled a "cooperative worker"	Separated from husband

6	162	2	Involutional psychotic depression	Thioridazine	Antidepressants	Mending-room worker; "dependable and pleasant worker"	Son died in Korean War; daughter committed suicide
7	106	None	Schizophrenia, paranoid	Chlorpromazine, then trifluoperazine, then perphenazine, then thioridazine	ECT		Father died (hospitalization precipitated by father's death)
8	95	1	Schizophrenia, catatonic; mild mental retardation	Trifluoperazine	ECT	Pressing-room worker; "works well"	Admitted from parent's home; discharged to sister
9	51	6	Schizophrenia, paranoid	Prochlorperazine	No	Hospital store; "good worker"	Lost contact with husband
10	44	3	Schizophrenia, chronic undifferentiated	Chlorpromazine plus trifluoperazine	No		Lost custody of oldest daughter
11	40	2	Schizophrenia, paranoid	Trifluoperazine	Antidepressants, ECT	Worked in hospital laundry	None known

TABLE 3. Hospitalization Index Circumstances (continued)

Case	Length of Hospital Stay (mos.)	Length of Psychotic Symptoms (mos.)	Length of Diagnosis	Time of Neuroleptics	Antidepressants and/or ECT	Off-Ward Job	Changes in Social Circumstances During Hospitalization
12	240	None	Schizophrenia, chronic undifferentiated; mild mental retardation	Trifluoperazine plus chlorpromazine	No	Ran cash register in employee cafeteria; "conscientious and competent"	Breakup of courtship relationship; loss of business; loss of family home; lost contact w/ siblings for 30 years
13	42	None	Depressive reaction; schizophrenia, catatonic	Trifluoperazine	Antidepressant, ECT		Lost contact with family
14	420	4	Schizophrenia, hebephrenic	Trifluoperazine	No	Worked in kitchen for 34 years	Lost contact with family; lost job
15	528	4	Schizophrenia, catatonic	Chlorpromazine	(Metrazol shock)	Housekeeping job; "hard worker"	Lost job; engagement broken
16	13	3	Schizophrenia	?	ECT (insulin coma)		Lost job
17	48	2	Psychotic depression; schizophrenia, paranoid; borderline mental retardation	Chlorpromazine, trifluoperazine	Antidepressant	Ward secretary	Lost position as domestic she had held for 15 yrs.; lost rights to visit her out-of-wedlock child placed with her sister

18	210	2	Schizophrenia, paranoid	Fluphenazine	ECT		Lost custody of her child and lost all contact with extended family including her child
19	188	None	Schizophrenia, paranoid	Chlorpromazine, trifluoperazine	ECT	Laundry; kitchen	Divorced; little contact with children
20	108	None	Schizophrenia, residual	Thioridazine	No	Housekeeping; "works diligently"	None known
21	124	None	Schizophrenia, chronic undifferentiated	Chlorpromazine	Antidepressant, ECT	Laundry worker; employed in hospital personnel office	Lost contact with 3 of 5 children
22	95	6	Schizophrenia, paranoid; epilepsy	Thiothixene	No	No known work (left hospital against medical advice)	Husband died during hospitalization; lost custody of all children
23	47	1	Schizophrenia, paranoid	Trifluoperazine, chlorpromazine	No	Housekeeping department	Rejected by siblings

TABLE 4. Follow-Up Circumstances

Case	Length of Follow-up (yr)	No. of Hospitalizations During Follow-up	Diagnosis in Outpatient Record	Medications	Proposed or Actual Decrease in Medications	Resistance to Medication Change	Tardive Dyskinesia (0–4)[a]	Social Adjustment
1	16	None	Schizophrenia, paranoid	Chlorpromazine, then fluphenazine decanoate	Yes	Agreeable	2	Worked full time; self-sufficient
2	7	None	Schizophrenia, chronic undifferentiated	Thioridazine	Yes	Indifferent	1	Lives in transitional residence; meets own needs
3	17	None	Schizophrenia, chronic undifferentiated	Trifluoperazine	Yes	Negative	2	Lives independently; part-time jobs and welfare
4	14	One	Schizophrenia, paranoid	Trifluoperazine, amitriptyline	Yes	Indifferent	0	Lives independently; has not been employed
5	19	One	Schizophrenia	Fluphenazine	Yes	Negative	2	Worked full-time; raised 7 children as a single parent
6	14	None	Schizophrenia, paranoid	Thioridazine, then chlorpromazine plus amitriptyline	Yes	Negative	1	Lives independently; very active in social community

154

7	17	None	Schizophrenia, paranoid	Thioridazine	Yes	Indifferent	0	Husband died 2 years after her discharge; she raises 4 sons alone and is employed out of the house
8	15	None	Schizophrenia, chronic undifferentiated	Trifluoperazine	Yes	Negative	1	Went from sister's to transitional living to living independently; works at Goodwill
9	23	One	Schizophrenia	Haloperidol, then chlorpromazine	Yes	Negative	0	Independent; employed as housekeeper and companion; executor of parent's will
10	16	two	Schizophrenia, paranoid	Fluphenazine decanoate plus chlorpromazine	Yes	Agreeable	1	Independent; works part time; provides child care for grandchildren
11	20	Two	Schizophrenia	Trifluoperazine plus chlorpromazine, then thioridazine	Yes	Negative	3	Functions well as wife and mother of 3 children
12	10	None	Schizophrenia, chronic undifferentiated	Trifluoperazine plus chlorpromazine	Yes	Negative	1	Lived independently with roommates and became their caretaker

TABLE 4. Follow-Up Circumstances (continued)

Case	Length of Follow-up (yr)	No. of Hospitalizations During Follow-up	Diagnosis in Outpatient Record	Medications	Proposed or Actual Decrease in Medications	Resistance to Medication Change	Tardive Dyskinesia (0–4)[a]	Social Adjustment
13	17	None	Schizophrenia, chronic undifferentiated	Trifluoperazine with and without imipramine	Yes	Negative	1	Graduated from business school; then worked as secretary; took care of ill parents
14	11	None	Schizophrenia, organic brain syndrome	Trifluoperazine, then haloperidol, then fluphenazine	Yes	Negative	2	Independent; not employed
15	9	None	Schizophrenia, residual	Chlorpromazine	Yes	Negative	1	Independent; full-time employment
16	33	One	Schizophrenia, residual; narcissistic personality disorder	Perphenazine, amitriptyline	Yes	Negative	0	Married after discharge; no children; volunteered 3 days per week at hospital
17	11	None	Schizophrenia; involutional depression	Perphenazine, amitriptyline	Yes	Negative	1	Independent; lived with roommates she cared for.
18	15	None	Schizophrenia, paranoid	Fluphenazine	Yes	Negative	3	Independent; became mother surrogate to group of college students; never worked

156

19	15	None	Schizophrenia, residual	Chlorpromazine	Yes	Negative	2	Independent; receives supplemental security income; very sociable
20	13	None	Schizophrenia, paranoid, in remission	Thioridazine	Yes	Negative	2	Has lived with same roommate since discharge; very social; assists in caring for a mentally retarded neighbor
21	15	None	Schizophrenia, residual	Chlorpromazine, thiothixene	No		0	Employed as state hospital laundry worker; reestablished contact with children; same roommate since 1971
22	15	None	Schizophrenia, chronic undifferentiated; mild mental retardation; seizure disorder; organic brain syndrome	Haloperidol	Yes	Indifferent	2	Lives in staffed residence; active social life
23	19	None	Schizoaffective disorder	Trifluoperazine, chlorpromazine, amitriptyline	Yes	Indifferent to neuroleptics; negative to antidepressants	2	Works sporadically as a janitor

[a] Global judgment of severity of abnormal movements on Abnormal Involuntary Movement Scale (item 8), scored 0-4.

We were able to document off-ward employment for 13 of the co-hort. Most of the patients had had major disruptions in their lives during the hospitalization, as detailed in Table 3.

Follow-up of the 22 women and 1 man is detailed in Table 4. The mean length of follow-up time was 15.5 years (range, 7–33 years). Sixteen women have had no psychiatric admissions since their discharge from the index hospitalization, four have had one, and two have had two. All the women had a schizophrenic diagnosis in their outpatient records, and all were still on a neuroleptic drug. Of the 21 women in whom decreases or discontinuation of medication had been suggested, 15 were opposed. Only five of the group had no evidence of tardive dyskinesia. Most of the group had lived independently.

Table 5 lists the *Diagnostic and Statistical Manual of Mental Disorders (Third Edition) (DSM-III; 8)* diagnoses we applied by reviewing the entire record. While 2 patients received diagnoses of schizophrenic disorders, 14 received Axis I diagnoses of affective disorders. Axis II diagnoses were made in five patients, one of whom had no Axis I diagnosis.

Discussion

Women in Institutions

Grob (9), in his essay, "Historical Origins of Deinstitutionalization," indicated that psychiatric institutions traditionally served two distinct groups of patients. One group benefited from brief confinement and then returned to functioning in the community; the other, with severe mental pathology, remained in the institution for longer times and then required "assistance." We have identified a third group who, like the first, benefited from brief confinement but who, like the second, remained in the institution for long periods. We have found this group to be made up predominantly of women. We turn now to attempts to understand this finding.

We do so, however, with caution. There is a long history in psychiatry of criticism of those who have attempted to understand gender differences in mental illness and its treatment. In 1844, Thurnam (10) told his colleagues, "The opinion which appears to have recently obtained that insanity is more prevalent amongst women than amongst men has, I believe, originated in an erroneous method of statistical analysis" (p 235). Wooley (11), in her 1910 discussion of the recent literature on the psychology of sex, indicated, "There is perhaps no field as aspiring to be scientific where flagrant personal bias, logic martyred in the cause of supporting a prejudice, unfounded assertions, and even sentimental rot and drivel, have run riot to such an extent as here" (p 340). And finally Pollitt, in the "Hers" column in the *New York Times* in 1986 remarked that "the history of psychiatry is a veritable riot of sexism" (12).

TABLE 5. *DSM-III* **Diagnosis by Case**

Case	Axis	Diagnosis
1	I.	Atypical paranoid disorder
2	I.	Major depression
	II.	Avoidant personality disorder
3	I.	Major depression
4	I.	Bipolar affective disorder (type II)
5	I.	Bipolar affective disorder
6	I.	Major depression
7	I.	Dysthymic disorder
	II.	Paranoid personality disorder
8	I.	Major depression
	II.	Schizoid personality disorder
	V Code.	Borderline intellectual function
9	I.	Bipolar affective disorder
10	I.	Schizophrenic disorder, paranoid subtype
11	I.	Schizoaffective disorder
12	I.	Conversion disorder
	II.	Dependent personality disorder
13	II.	Passive-aggressive personality disorder
14	I.	Schizophreniform disorder
15	I.	Acute paranoid disorder
16	I.	Major depression
17	I.	Major depression
18	I.	Major depression
19	I.	Major depression
20	I.	Bipolar affective disorder
21	I.	Major depression
22	I.	Atypical organic brain syndrome; mild mental retardation
	III.	Seizure disorder
23	I.	Alcohol hallucinosis; dysthymic disorder; alcohol dependence

TABLE 6. Admissions (1940–1985) and Discharges (1959–1985) by Sex, Mayview State Hospital

Year	No. of Admissions			No. of Discharges		
	Male	Female	Ratio of Males/Females	Male	Female	Ratio of Males/Females
1940	355	296	1.20			
1941	295	309	0.95			
1942	257	257	1.00			
1943	268	244	1.10			
1944	290	291	1.00			
1945	252	279	0.90			
1946	326	318	1.03			
1947	368	359	1.03			
1948	442	410	1.08			
1949	443	399	1.11			
1950	470	412	1.14			
1951	477	431	1.11			
1952	431	418	1.03			
1953	394	346	1.14			
1954	417	385	1.08			
1955	363	381	0.95			
1956	366	393	0.93			
1957	360	434	0.83			
1958	498	478	1.04			
1959	397	380	1.04	401	365	1.10
1960	442	430	1.03	393	382	1.03
1961	407	442	0.92	497	438	1.13
1962	433	389	1.11	367	369	0.99

Year						
1963	261	255	1.02	418	295	1.42
1964	527	385	1.37	479	345	1.39
1965	474	357	1.33	519	356	1.46
1966	447	341	1.31	512	367	1.40
1967	479	347	1.38	491	398	1.23
1968	413	277	1.49	422	336	1.26
1969	427	279	1.53	635	643	0.99
1970	437	317	1.38	622	562	1.11
1971	530	349	1.52	796	706	1.13
1972	510	372	1.37	510	369	1.38
1973	396	316	1.25	425	365	1.16
1974	289	235	1.23	426	379	1.12
1975	260	235	1.11	302	299	1.01
1976	288	219	1.32	340	314	1.08
1977	330	219	1.51	385	257	1.50
1978	474	239	1.98	441	282	1.56
1979	476	298	1.60	500	299	1.67
1980	383	208	1.84	410	275	1.49
1981	447	209	2.14	503	247	2.04
1982	476	258	1.84	494	270	1.83
1983	494	251	1.97	335	540	0.62
1984	574	353	1.63	605	387	1.56
1985	574	355	1.62	585	399	1.47
Total	18,717	15,155	1.24[a]	12,813	10,244	1.25[a]

[a]Mean ratio of males/females.

161

We proceed because, like Stone (13), we are concerned that "perhaps the most penetrating and convincing attack on the hidden and destructive values in psychiatry has related to the subject of women" (p 891).

Differential Prevalence of Mental Illness

If there is more mental illness in women than in men, and there are more female admissions than male admissions to psychiatric facilities, or both, the gender distribution in our cohort of patients could simply reflect the population from which they came. The belief that women are more mentally ill than men was reported by Gove and associates (13–16) and investigated by the President's Commission on Mental Health (17). Chesler (18) documented the fact that more women than men have been institutionalized in psychiatric facilities. The findings leading to this body of literature, however, have been extensively discussed and attacked during the past 10 years (19–23).

To determine if the gender distribution of our results paralleled the regional inpatient institutional population, we examined admissions by gender since 1940 and discharges by gender since 1959 (earliest data available) from the catchment area state hospital. As shown in Table 6, women represent fewer than 50 percent of the admissions and discharges for those years.

While the absolute numbers of male and female patients may not account for our finding, the gender distribution in certain diagnostic categories might have produced populations of women more at risk for the pattern of treatment we have defined. Schizophrenia was the diagnosis given to most patients who met our criteria during their index hospitalizations. Seeman (24–26), Lewine and colleagues (27–29), and Flor-Henry (30, 31), among others (32–36), have indicated that schizophrenia in women is distinct from schizophrenia in men. Although this position has its detractors (37, 38), there is good evidence that women with schizophrenia in general have a later onset, better premorbid functioning, more affectively colored symptoms, a better response to treatment, and a better prognosis than do men with schizophrenia. The mean age at first hospitalization of women in our population who were diagnosed as having schizophrenia was 32.4 years old, suggesting a later onset. The difference in the nature of schizophrenia in women and the probability of a greater prevalence of schizophrenia in women than in men (39) would produce a group of schizophrenic women vulnerable to the treatment history we have documented without a comparable group of schizophrenic men vulnerable to this treatment history.

A similar argument might be made for affective disorders. In our application of *DSM-III* diagnostic groups to the hospital records, we determined that a preponderance of the patients suffered from affective disorders. Whether this reflects the historic overdiagnosis of schizophrenia and underdiagnosis of affective disorders in the United States (40, 41), or whether this supports Lewine's contention that schizophrenia in women is often atypical and characterized by prominent affective symptoms (28), is an open question. Nonetheless, the female predominance in the lifetime prevalence of depression (39, 42–45) might also produce a group vulnerable to the treatment we have documented, a group with a disproportionate number of women.

The overrepresentation of women in certain diagnostic groups and the characteristics of the pathology in these groups might make women more likely to experience prolonged institutional stays and prolonged neuroleptic treatment. However, there are other contributing causes. To understand why women are especially vulnerable to the above-described treatment history, we turn from the examination of diseases per se to what Goffman (46) has called "contingencies."

Women's Roles in the Community

Two ways in which women's functioning in society have traditionally been differentiated from men's may partially account for the prolonged institutional stays of women in our cohort. The first of these is economic (10, 47–49). Rushing indicated that "the continued hospitalization of middle-aged males is more disruptive to others, economically and organizationally, than is the continued hospitalization of most middle-aged females" (49, p 212). Middle-aged women would therefore have longer stays than middle-aged men because pressure for return to the community would be less intense. Rushing found this to be the case in his study of all first admissions to Tennessee state mental hospitals between 1956 and

1965 (49). Howard and Howard (47) also found this in their analysis of National Institute of Mental Health data for the United States. The second way to account for the prolonged stays of women is based on their role as "nurturers." Articles published in the 1980s have repeatedly indicated that women occupy the nurturant role (16, 50–53) and are, by and large, "the caretakers of the mentally ill" (52). Therefore, a woman at home in the preliberation era might have been more likely to be prepared for the return of her ex-patient husband than a man might have been to minister to his ex-patient wife.

Sex-Role Stereotyping and the Resultant Catch-22 in the Institution

During the past 15 years, the literature on sex-role stereotyping and its relationship to psychiatric treatment has been extensive and not without controversy (21, 34, 44, 54–67). The classic work in this field is that of Broverman and associates (54, 55), who found:

> clinicians are more likely to suggest that healthy women differ from healthy men by being more submissive, less independent, less adventurous, more easily influenced, less aggressive, less competitive, more excitable in minor crises, having their feelings more easily hurt, being more emotional, more concerned about their appearances, less objective, and disliking math and science. This constellation seems a most unusual way of describing any mature, healthy individual. (54, p 4, 5)

Kaplan has succinctly summarized Broverman and associates' work as follows:

> ... To be considered an unhealthy adult, women must act as women are supposed to act (conform too much to the female sex role stereotype); to be considered an unhealthy woman, women must act as men are supposed to act (not conform enough to the female sex-role stereotype). ... This Catch-22 predicts that women are bound to be labeled unhealthy one way or another. ... (63, p 788)

Broverman and associates' findings have been echoed by Carmen and associates in a review article in the *American Journal of Psychiatry*: "Submissiveness, compliance, passivity, helplessness, weakness have been encouraged in women and incorporated into some prevalent psychological theories" (44, p 1321).

American psychiatric institutions in the mid-twentieth century actually provided a context within which there was no way out for better-functioning women. If a woman deviated from sex-role expectations by being aggressive, assertive, independent, or direct, or by lobbying vigorously for discharge, she was seen as requiring treatment for her pathology and therefore needing a longer stay. If she conformed to sex-role stereotypes and was quiet, neat, gentle, or tactful, who in the busy, overcrowded, understaffed institution was going to get around to reviewing her treatment or to discharging her? Moreover, if her role conformity allowed her to function well in a job necessary for the running of the institution (note the institutional work histories of the women in our sample), what member of the institution's staff would want to discharge her?

Institutions and the Ideal Patient

Although there is controversy about the effects of gender on the length of institutional residence (18, 48, 68), comprehending the interface between typification of women and institutional needs adds to our understanding of why the particular women described in this chapter had such prolonged stays.

Women are more comfortable than men in roles requiring them to be passive (47, 69), compliant (70), dependent (71, 72), submissive (69, 71), and to conform to the environment (71). Expressed anger by women is often viewed as inappropriate (44, 70, 72), and hence women are easier to exploit (70). These characteristics contribute to Chesler's notion that "perhaps one of the reasons women embark and re-embark on 'psychiatric careers' more than men do is because they feel, quite horribly, at 'home within them' " (18, p 35).

Descriptions of the patient role in the psychiatric hospital of the 1950s and 1960s illustrate why women would be the preferred patients. Stanton and Schwartz reported that "a patient has to learn, and in some way to conform to, the rules, restrictions, and freedoms of the hospital. . . . He must submit in some way to the power of the staff" (73, p 170). Dunham and Weinberg indicated that "the attendants . . . function to inhibit any normal assertiveness, any emerging interests or any reasonable expression of desires which patients may have" (74, p 248). And Levinson and Gallagher believed that "the ideal patient ... is eager to comply with the rules and to maintain harmonious but relatively affectless relationships with staff and other patients" (75, p 219).

The women in our cohort come even closer to the definition of the preferred patient because they are less debilitated and have a higher level of functioning than most. Levinson and Gallagher called the ideal patient "a person who has had a nervous breakdown but is not really crazy" (75). Braginsky and associates demonstrated that patients who became "workers" early in their hospitalization remained in the facility longer than others (76). And Weinstein concluded that less-ill patients were more positive about their hospitalization than those more severely disturbed (77).

Hence, the women in our cohort approximate the ideal candidates for prolonged stay: conforming workers who were without prolonged psychosis, would be no management problem, and would contribute to the functioning of the institution.

Illness Behavior and Follow-Up

It has generally been reported that women use outpatient psychiatric treatment services more than men (20, 78). This may be due in large measure to the observations, made repeatedly, that mental illness in one's own person is more acceptable to women than to men; that the sick role is more compatible with women's functioning in society than with men's; and that help-seeking is more acceptable to women than to men (35, 71, 79–82).

In the CDC population as a whole 54 percent of the patients are women. It is noteworthy that of those patients older than 55, 80 (82 percent) are women. Of these, 19 are part of our cohort.

It is possible that the women in our cohort became differentiated from their male counterparts not during institutionalization, but rather at follow-up. While we believe this to be unlikely, the small percentage of male patients in the CDC population over age 55 is intriguing. Segal and Everett-Dille (82), in a study of former mental patients living in sheltered-care facilities in California, stated, "it appears ... that, unlike men, women who have spent large amounts of time in state mental hospitals want out of the mental health care system totally" (p 17). This does not seem to be the case in the CDC, where the older deinstitutionalized population is predominantly female.

It is possible that there are men with characteristics similar to those of the study cohort who are simply not in treatment in the CDC. If they exist, we can at best speculate that they may be living in the community without treatment, or that they may be largely treated by the Veterans Administration, or that they may have had a greater mortality than age-matched women. While we do not believe that differential rates or loci of follow-up by gender account for our findings, the overrepresentation of older women in the clinic population as a whole remains an incompletely explained finding.

Women and Neuroleptics

Our findings led us to speculate on the reasons that women with brief psychotic episodes might be prescribed neuroleptics in the first place. In general, studies have shown that women are much more likely than men to be prescribed psychotropic medications. This is thought to be the result of a cultural fit between women's attitudes toward themselves and physicians' attitudes toward women (83, 84).

Once neuroleptic drugs have been prescribed, can we understand why women continue to take them? Several studies of schizophrenic patients show that women do better than men on neuroleptics: Women have more symptomatic improvement and are less likely to relapse (85–87). Why this is so is unclear, but women tend to have better compliance with medication, and they tend to have better therapeutic relationships (24).

The long-term use of neuroleptic drugs produces a range of potential morbidities. The most prominent of these is tardive dyskinesia (TD). Indeed, 40 percent of our study cohort have significant movement abnormalities, with 35 percent meeting proposed research diagnostic criteria for probable TD (88). This prevalence rate is the same as that in the entire outpatient clinic. On the whole, this finding is not surprising and certainly supports other documentation that TD develops in patients with a variety of psychiatric diagnoses (89). Based on the nature of the cohort, we might have suspected an even higher prevalence of TD than was found. There is some evidence that TD is more prevalent in women than in men, that prevalence of TD clearly increases with the age of the sample population, and that patients with affective disorders appear to be at higher risk for developing TD than schizophrenic patients (89, 90).

Thus this older, female, affectively disordered group appears at high risk for developing TD.

A hypothesized risk from long-term neuroleptic treatment is the limbic equivalent of TD, which has been variously called tardive psychosis, tardive dysmentia, tardive dysphrenia, and supersensitivity psychosis (91–94). Based on the concept that TD is the result of dopamine supersensitivity in the nigrostriatum, various investigators have suggested that a similar supersensitivity might develop in the mesolimbic system and result in a supersensitivity psychosis or other behavioral changes. As described by Chouinard and Jones (94) supersensitivity psychosis would be expected to have pharmacologic characteristics similar to those of TD. Thus, psychotic symptoms would appear shortly after neuroleptics were discontinued or decreased in patients with significant neuroleptic exposure.

While it remains unclear that supersensitivity psychosis actually develops as described (95), the patients in this cohort are an ideal group to investigate. Davis and Rosenberg (96) have noted, "Patients who are not schizophrenic but who have chronically received neuroleptic medications ... can provide information on the possible induction of mesolimbic dopamine receptors supersensitivity. These non-schizophrenic patients might develop schizophrenic symptoms upon discontinuation of long-term neuroleptic treatment."

Wilson and associates (92) recently described a condition resulting from long-term neuroleptic use that they call tardive dysmentia. They observed that clearly schizophrenic patients develop behavioral changes after years of neuroleptic treatment that make them appear more affectively disturbed. These behavioral changes include loudness and loquaciousness, a prevailing euphoric mood with marked lability, and an overly close approach to the examiner. These characteristics do not seem to typify the study cohort. Nor can tardive dysmentia account for the changes in diagnosis of the study cohort to predominantly affective disorders, since these changes are based on reviewing the entire clinical history.

Our study population is similar to the population of overly compliant patients described by Lesser and Friedman (97) who resist medication reduction as the result of their conviction that such changes will result in recurrence of illness. Although, in fact, schizophrenic patients do have an obvious increased risk of relapse if medication is stopped or decreased, such decompensations are usually not immediate and occur most often several months following a dose change (86). Yet our study patients often maintain that they get ill immediately after dose reduction. Lesser and Friedman (97) suggested that medications meet patients' unconscious oral-dependency needs and as such cannot be safely removed without "substituting other forms of nurturance."

There are, in addition, pharmacologic explanations for increasing symptomatology immediately after neuroleptic dose reduction or discontinuation. Autonomic and behavioral withdrawal symptoms, which can be mistaken for early symptoms of relapse, have been documented since the late 1950s (98). Symptoms occur within days to one week of the medication change and disappear by the end of two weeks and include nausea, vomiting, diarrhea, perspiration, restlessness, insomnia, rhinorrhea, headache, increased appetite, and giddiness (99). In their review of neuroleptic withdrawal syndromes, Gardos and associates (99) postulated that these symptoms may be due to cholinergic rebound and occur most often with low-potency, highly anticholinergic drugs like chlorpromazine and thioridazine. Women may be more prone than men to develop these withdrawal symptoms (99). Chouinard and associates (100) recently found a high proportion of patients rapidly developing insomnia, anxiety, and restlessness while being gradually switched from low- to high-potency neuroleptics. They concluded that these withdrawal symptoms can lead to overcompliance with low-potency neuroleptics (which were being taken by 50 percent of our cohort) and difficulty achieving minimal effective dose.

In summary, once on neuroleptic drugs, chronically treated patients like those in our sample may have a number of reasons for wanting to stay on psychotropic medication, including a fear of relapse of the underlying disease (patients in our sample uniformly recall Dr. X's warning them never to stop their drugs lest they become "crazy again"), an experience with supersensitivity psychoses, a dependence on pills for sustenance, and a wish to avoid uncomfortable withdrawal symptoms. When medication is reduced and the patient feels worse, she returns to the clinic and says, "I told you so. I need that Thorazine."

Implications for the Future

In view of the fact that state hospitals have largely been depopulated and community treatment has become the norm, are our observations of more than historical interest? We believe they are.

The cohort we have identified constitutes a naturalistic experiment. We are being offered a unique opportunity to study the effects of the chronic administration of neuroleptic medication without concurrent schizophrenia. We suggest that patients such as those we have described be identified at multiple sites, be followed in controlled clinical settings, and then undergo postmortem examinations.

While deinstitutionalization has remained the thrust of public-sector psychiatry in the 1980s, there are those who now call for providing patients "asylum" (101–103) and others who carry this to the point of wanting to resurrect "asylums" (104–106). Psychiatric practitioners need to attend specifically to the needs of women and the potential to misperceive those needs in any contemplated changes in the loci of treatment for the chronically mentally ill.

The chronically mentally ill in the community are often less "deinstitutionalized" than they are "transinstitutionalized." Halfway houses, board-and-care residences, supervised apartments, nursing homes, and the like are just as vulnerable to prolonging dependency and to treating women labeled chronically mentally ill inappropriately as were the state hospitals. We should add this phenomenon to Bachrach's list of the consequences of public policy in the deinstitutionalization of women (107). The women we have described are ideal residents of community programs, and we need to examine whether or not their stays are prolonged beyond their needs because it is easier to serve them than it is to serve newly discharged patients, young adult chronic patients, or the homeless mentally ill.

We should be reminded of the tenacity of psychiatric labeling and how that labeling translates into treatment. The women in our cohort, once diagnosed schizophrenic, kept that label despite documentation in the outpatient record of its inappropriateness. We have prolonged mistreatment and we continue to do so.

Finally, our study documents a classic example of sexism in psychiatry. We can only hope that psychiatric treatment of women in institutions of the future will not repeat the iatrogenic creation of psychiatric chronicity in women.

References

1. Fuller R: An Account of the Imprisonment and Suffering of Robert Fuller of Cambridge. Boston, 1833.
2. Stone ET: A Sketch of the Life of Elizabeth T. Stone, and her Persecutions, with an Appendix of Her Treatment and Sufferings While in the Charlestown McLean Asylum, Where She Was Confined with the Pretense of Insanity. Printed for the author, 1842
3. Packard EPW: Modern Persecution, or Married Woman's Liabilities, vol II. Hartford, CT, 1874
4. Lunt ATP: Behind Bars. Boston, Lee and Shepard, 1871
5. Lee K: A Year at Elgin Asylum. New York, Irving Co., 1902
6. Jefferson L: These Are My Sisters. Tulsa, OK, Vickers Publishing Co., 1947
7. Rose: Mad people are revolutionaries. Madness Network News 7:4, 1985
8. American Psychiatric Association. Diagnostic and Statistical Manual of Mental Disorders (Third Edition). Washington, DC, American Psychiatric Association, 1980.
9. Grob GN: Historical origins of deinstitutionalization, in Deinstitutionalization: New Directions for Mental Health Services No. 17. Edited by Bachrach LL. San Francisco, Jossey-Bass, 1983
10. Thurnam J: On the relative liability of the two sexes to insanity. Am J Insanity 3:235–245, 1846
11. Wooley HT: Psychological literature. A review of the recent literature on the psychology of sex. Psychol Bull 7:335–342, 1910
12. Pollitt K: Hers. New York Times, 9 January 1986, p 16
13. Stone AA: Presidential address: conceptual ambiguity and morality in modern psychiatry. Am J Psychiatry 137:887–891, 1980
14. Gove WR, Tudor JF: Adult sex roles and mental illness. Am J Sociol 78:812–835, 1973

15. Clancy K, Gove W: Sex differences in mental illness: an analysis of response bias in self-reports. Am J Sociol 80:205–216, 1974
16. Gove WR: Gender differences in mental and physical illness: the effects of fixed roles and nuturant roles. Soc Sci Med 19:77–91, 1984
17. President's Commission on Mental Health: Report of the Subpanel on the Mental Health of Women, in Report to the President, vol 3. Washington, DC, US Government Printing Office, 1978.
18. Chesler P: Women and Madness. New York, Doubleday, 1972
19. Dohrenwald BP, Dohrenwald BS: Sex differences and psychiatric disorders. Am J Sociol 81:1447–1454, 1976
20. Belle D: Who uses mental health facilities?, in The Mental Health of Women. Edited by Guttenag M, Salasin S, Belle D. New York, Academic Press, 1980
21. Sherman JA: Therapist attitudes and sex-role stereotyping, in Women and Psychotherapy. Edited by Brodsky AM, Hare-Mustin R. New York, Guilford Press, 1980
22. Al-Issa I: Gender and adult psychopathology, in Gender and Psychopathology. Edited by Al-Issa I. New York, Academic Press, 1982
23. Busfield J: Gender and mental illness. Int J Ment Health 11:46–66, 1982
24. Seeman MV: Gender differences in schizophrenics. Can J Psychiatry 27:107–112, 1982
25. Seeman MV: Schizophrenic men and women require different treatment programs. Journal of Psychiatric Treatment and Evaluation 5:143–148, 1983
26. Seeman MV: Sex and schizophrenia. Can J Psychiatry 30:313–315, 1985
27. Lewine RRJ: Sex differences in schizophrenia: a commentary. Schizophr Bull 5:4–7, 1979
28. Lewine RRJ: Sex differences in schizophrenia: timing or subtype. Psychol Bull 90:432–444, 1981
29. Burbach DJ, Lewine R, Meltzer HY: Diagnostic concordance for schizophrenia as a function of sex. J Consult Clin Psychol 52:478–479, 1984
30. Flor-Henry P: Psychosis, neurosis and epilepsy. Br J Psychiatry 124:144–150, 1974

31. Flor-Henry P: Schizophrenia: sex differences. Can J Psychiatry 30:319–322, 1985
32. Raskin A, Golob R: Occurrence of sex and social class differences in premorbid competence, symptom and outcome measures in acute schizophrenia. Psychol Rep 18:11–22, 1966
33. Test MA, Berlin SB: Issues of special concern to chronically mentally ill women. Professional Psychology 12:136–145, 1981
34. Al-Issa I: Gender and schizophrenia, in Gender and Psychopathology. Edited by Al-Issa I. New York, Academic Press, 1982
35. Salokangas RKR: Prognostic implications of the sex of schizophrenic patients. Br J Psychiatry 142:145–151, 1983
36. LaTorre RA: Schizophrenia, in Sex Roles and Psychopathology. Edited by Widom CS. New York, Plenum, 1984
37. Leventhal DB, Schuck JR, Rothstein H: Gender differences in schizophrenia. J Nerv Ment Dis 172:464–467, 1984
38. Loyd D, Simpson JC, Tsuang MT: Are there sex differences in the long-term outcome of schizophrenia? J Nerv Ment Dis 173:643–649, 1985
39. Robins LN, Helzer JE, Weisman MM, et al: Lifetime prevalence of specific psychiatric disorders in three sites. Arch Gen Psychiatry 41:949–958, 1984
40. Taylor MA, Abrams R: The prevalence of schizophrenia: a reassessment using modern diagnostic criteria. Am J Psychiatry 135:945–948, 1978
41. Lipton AA, Simon FS: Psychiatric diagnosis in a state hospital: Manhattan State revisited. Hosp Comm Psychiatry 36:368–373, 1985
42. Seiden AM: Overview: research on the psychology of women. II. Women in families, work, and psychotherapy. Am J Psychiatry 133:1111–1123, 1976
43. Weisman MM, Klerman GL: Sex differences and the epidemiology of depression. Arch Gen Psychiatry 34:98–111, 1977
44. Carmen E, Russo NF, Miller JB: Inequality and women's mental health: an overview. Am J Psychiatry 138:1319–1330, 1981
45. Jenkins R, Clare AW: Women and mental illness. Br Med J 291:1521–1522, 1985

46. Goffman E: Asylums. Garden City, NY, Doubleday, 1961
47. Howard EM, Howard JL: Women in institutions: treatment in prisons and mental hospitals, in Women in Therapy. Edited by Franks V, Burtle V. New York, Brunner/Mazel, 1974
48. Tudor W, Tudor JF, Gove WR: The effect of sex role differences on the social control of mental illness. J Health Soc Behav 18:98–112, 1977
49. Rushing WA: The functional importance of sex roles and sex-related behavior in societal reactions to residual deviance. J Health Soc Behav 20:208–217, 1979
50. Vanfossen BE: Sex differences in the mental health effects of spouse support and equity. J Health Soc Behav 22:130–143, 1981
51. Belle D: The stress of caring: women as providers of social support, in Handbook of Stress. Edited by Goldberger L, Breznitz S. New York, Free Press, 1982
52. Thurer SL: Deinstitutionalization and women: where the buck stops. Hosp Community Psychiatry 34:1162–1163, 1983
53. Kessler RC, McLeon JD: Sex differences in vulnerability to undesirable life events. American Sociological Review 49:620–631, 1984
54. Broverman IK, Broverman DM, Clarkson FE, et al: Sex-role stereotypes and clinical judgments of mental health. J Consult Clin Psychol 34:1–7, 1970
55. Broverman IK, Vogel SR, Broverman DM, et al: Sex-role stereotypes: a current appraisal. Journal of Social Issues 28:59–78, 1972
56. Lerner HE: Early origins of envy and devaluation of women: implications for sex role stereotypes. Bull Menninger Clin 38:538–543, 1974
57. Levine SV, Kamin LE, Levine EL: Sexism and psychiatry. Am J Orthopsychiatry 44:327–336, 1974
58. Doherty EG: Are differential discharge criteria used for men and women psychiatric inpatients? J Health Soc Behav 9:107–116, 1978
59. Zeldow PB: Sex differences in psychiatric evaluation and treatment. Arch Gen Psychiatry 35:89–93, 1978
60. Abramowitz CV, Dokecki PR: The politics of clinical judgment: early empirical returns. Psychol Bull 84:460–476, 1977

61. King E: Sex bias in psychoactive drug advertisements. Psychiatry 43:129–137, 1980
62. Rosenfield S: Sex roles and societal reactions to mental illness: the labeling of "deviant" deviance. J Health Soc Behav 23:18–24, 1982
63. Kaplan M: A woman's view of DSM-III. Am Psychologist 38:786–792, 1983
64. Widom CS: Sex roles and psychopathology, in Sex Roles and Psychopathology. Edited by Widom CS. New York, Plenum, 1984
65. Zeldow PB: Sex roles, psychological assessment, and patient management, in Sex Roles and Psychopathology. Edited by Widom CS. New York, Plenum, 1984
66. American Psychological Association: Developing a National Agenda to Address Women's Mental Health Needs. Washington, DC, American Psychological Association, 1985
67. Weisman CS, Teitelbaum MA: Physician gender and the physician-patient relationship: recent evidence and relevant questions. Soc Sci Med 20:1119–1127, 1985
68. Burvill PW, Mittelman: A follow-up study of chronic mental hospital patients 1959–1969. Soc Psychiatry 6:167–171, 1971
69. Greenberg RP, Fisher S, Shapiro J: Sex-role development and response to medication by psychiatric in-patients. Psychol Rep 33:675–677, 1973
70. Seiden AM: Overview: research on the psychology of women. I. Gender difference and sexual and reproductive life. Am J Psychiatry 133:995–1007, 1976
71. Garai JE: Sex differences in mental health. Genet Psychol Monogr 81:123–142, 1970
72. Abernethy V: Cultural perspectives on the impact of women's changing roles on psychiatry. Am J Psychiatry 133:657–661, 1976
73. Stanton AH, Schwartz MS: The Mental Hospital. New York, Basic Books, 1954
74. Dunham HW, Weinberg SK: The Culture of the State Mental Hospital. Detroit, Wayne State University Press, 1960
75. Levinson DJ, Gallagher EB: Patienthood in the Mental Hospital. Boston, Houghton Mifflin, 1964
76. Braginsky BM, Braginsky DD, Ring K: Methods of Madness. New York, Holt, Rinehart and Winston, 1969

77. Weinstein RM: Patient attitudes toward mental hospitalization: a review of quantitative research. J Health Soc Behav 20:237–258, 1979
78. Russo NF, Sobel SB: Sex differences in the utilization of mental health facilities. Professional Psychology 12:7–19, 1981
79. Phillips DL: Rejection of the mentally ill: the influence of behavior and sex. American Sociological Review 29:679–687, 1964
80. Nathanson CA: Illness and the feminine role: a theoretical review. Soc Sci Med 9:57–62, 1975
81. Horwitz A: The pathways into psychiatric treatment: some differences between men and women. J Health Soc Behav 18:169–178, 1977
82. Segal SP, Everett-Dille L: Coping styles and factors in male/female social integration. Acta Psychiatr Scand 61:8–20, 1980
83. Fidell LS: Sex differences in psychotropic drug use. Professional Psychology 12:156–162, 1981
84. Cooperstock R: Sex differences in psychotropic drug use. Soc Sci Med 12B:179–186, 1978
85. Goldberg SC, Schooler NR, Davidson EM, et al: Sex and race differences in response to drug treatment among schizophrenics. Psychopharmacologia 9:31–47, 1966
86. Hogarty GE, Goldberg SC, Schooler NR, et al: Drug and sociotherapy in the aftercare of schizophrenic patients: II. 2-year relapse rates. Arch Gen Psychiatry 31:603–608, 1974
87. Goldstein MJ, Rodnick, EH, Evans JR, et al: Drug and family therapy in the aftercare of acute schizophrenics. Arch Gen Psychiatry 35:1169–1177, 1978
88. Schooler NR, Kane JM: Research diagnoses for tardive dyskinesia. Arch Gen Psychiatry 39:486–487, 1982
89. Kane JM, Smith JM: Tardive dyskinesia: prevalence and risk factors, 1959 to 1979. Arch Gen Psychiatry 39:473–481, 1982
90. Kane JM, Woerder M, Borenstein N, et al: Integrating incidence and prevalence of tardive dyskinesia. Presented at the IVth World Congress of Biological Psychiatry. Philadelphia, 8–13 September 1985
91. McCarthy JJ: "Tardive psychosis." Am J Psychiatry 135:625–626, 1978
92. Wilson IC, Garbutt JC, Lanier CF, et al: Is there a tardive dysmentia? Schizophr Bull 9:187–192, 1983

93. Forrest DV, Fahn S: Tardive dysphrenia and subjective akathisia. J Clin Psychiatry 40:206, 1979
94. Chouinard G, Jones BD: Neuroleptic-induced supersensitivity psychosis: clinical and pharmacologic characteristics. Am J Psychiatry 137:16–21, 1980
95. Weinberger DR, Bigelow LB, Klein ST, et al: Drug withdrawal in chronic schizophrenic patients: in search of neuroleptic-induced supersensitivity psychosis. J Clin Psychopharmacol 1:120–123, 1981
96. Davis KL, Rosenberg GS: Is there a limbic system equivalent of tardive dyskinesia? Biol Psychiatry 14:699–703, 1979
97. Lesser IM, Friedman CTH: Attitudes toward medication change among chronically impaired psychiatric patients. Am J Psychiatry 138:801–803, 1981
98. Brooks GW: Withdrawal from neuroleptic drugs. Am J Psychiatry 115:931–932, 1959
99. Gardos G, Cole JO, Tarsy D: Withdrawal syndromes associated with antipsychotic drugs. Am J Psychiatry 135:1321–1324, 1978
100. Chouinard G, Bradwejn J, Annable L, et al: Withdrawal symptoms after long-term treatment with low-potency neuroleptics. J Clin Psychiatry 45:500–502, 1984
101. Bachrach LL: Asylum and chronically ill psychiatric patients. Am J Psychiatry 141:975–978, 1984
102. Lamb HR, Peele R: The need for continuing asylum and sanctuary. Hosp Community Psychiatry 35:798–802, 1984
103. Talbott JA: The need for asylum, not asylums. Hosp Community Psychiatry 35:209, 1984
104. Sigel GS: In defense of state hospitals. Hosp Community Psychiatry 35:1234–1235, 1984
105. Gralnick A: Build a better state hospital: deinstitutionalization has failed. Hosp Community Psychiatry 36:738–741, 1985
106. Gritter GW: State hospitals. Psychiatric News 21(1):2, 20, 1986 (letter)
107. Bachrach LL: Deinstitutionalization and women. Am Psychologist 39:1171–1177, 1984

Chapter 11

Chronically Mentally Ill Women: Conclusions

CAROL C. NADELSON, M.D.

Chapter 11

Chronically Mentally Ill Women: Conclusions

*T*his volume evolved from an invitational Presidential Sympo-
sium held at the May 1986 Annual Meeting of the American Psychiatric Association. It is the first time that data from a variety of
sources have delineated existing gender differences in the experiences and needs of those with chronic mental illness. The authors
have amply demonstrated that research in mental illness often ig-
nores such differences. This oversight leads to the development of
generic clinical programs that do not attend to gender-related needs,
to differences in the course and outcome of illness, or to differences
in the care available to men and to women.

In her introductory chapter, Dr. Bachrach emphasizes that, in
addition to the disabilities experienced by virtue of their illnesses,
chronically mentally ill women have additional gender-specific difficulties that are generated by societal responses to these women.
Since, as Dr. Bachrach points out, women constitute nearly two-
thirds of the population of the chronically mentally ill in the United
States, it is essential "that the vestiges of stereotyped thinking about
their service needs be eliminated; that discriminatory practices,
whether they are intended or not, be removed; and that planning
within the system of care be adapted to meet the special needs of
this service population."

Dr. Seeman cites recent evidence that men and women do, in
fact, differ in their responses to medication, as well as in other variables. Women have a later onset of schizophrenia, and Dr. Seeman
speculates that this may protect them against chronicity. She notes
that maintenance doses of neuroleptics are lower in early adulthood
for women, and only become higher later in life. Thus, postmeno-
pausal women may be more prone to late-developing side effects.
The role of estrogen and brain laterality are important in understanding gender differences in major mental illness.

Dr. Seeman also considers the context of treatment, including available ancillary services such as vocational training, child care, and housing. The availability of these services has an important influence on medication response and illness outcome. Likewise, she emphasizes the importance of clinicians' attitudes and values, since they affect the course of chronic mental illness in women.

The various points raised by Dr. Seeman take on added significance in view of the so-called "greying of America." The expected increase in the number of elderly persons will include disproportionately more women. Many of them will be chronic mental patients. Their needs will be important to consider in planning future health care delivery in the United States.

Dr. Bennett and associates point to yet another kind of gender difference that must be taken into account. They indicate that there are different behavioral expressions of illness for men and women. The male patients they studied, in an institutional setting, showed a pattern of more physically and sexually threatening and assaultive behavior, whereas the women showed more self-destructive, verbally assaultive, and generally nonviolent but irritating behaviors. Thus, these authors confirm earlier reports that stereotypical contrasts in male-female behavioral patterns are preserved in the population of chronically mentally ill patients. We can expect that responses to these behaviors, as well as to deviations from them, may affect the course of illness. The types and levels of resources provided may also be affected by how troublesome patients are to those responsible for their care.

While Lewine (1) has reported that hospitalized schizophrenic women are more agitated and aggressive, less social, and less manageable than hospitalized schizophrenic men, it is likely that this observation reflects differences in specific hospitalization patterns and practices. Lewine has suggested that schizophrenic women with negative behavioral characteristics were more likely to be hospitalized than those who were more tractable and unaggressive. Since male subjects predominate in studies of chronic mental illness, many of the gender differences that may emerge if we reverse dependent and independent variables in our studies are obscured. Indeed, the fact that female schizophrenics are more often characterized by better premorbid competence, later onset of illness, and an atypical pattern of symptom development reinforces the difficulty of understanding gender differences (2).

Dr. Goering and colleagues turn to still another variable by emphasizing the role of work in the lives of chronically mentally ill women. They point out how often this issue is ignored for women, despite the fact that women continue to fulfill their multiple obligations and to function, despite serious illness.

Ms. Leighton's first-person account of her experience with severe mental illness and hospitalization adds a perspective often lacking in professional discussions. Her eloquent statement points to directions for planning treatment and long-term care that are often ignored and that service providers would do well to heed.

The chapters by Dr. Bachrach and Dr. Handel, reprinted from *Hospital and Community Psychiatry*, were chosen to fill out our exploration of the problems of chronically mentally ill women. Dr. Bachrach elucidates the need for program development for these patients, and she addresses three specific areas—homelessness, skills training, and family planning—emphasizing the need to avoid generic reproductionism in program planning. In her emphasis on the need for comprehensive care, Dr. Handel provides disquieting data on the extent to which pelvic examinations are deferred or omitted for mentally ill women, reminding us of our responsibilities to these patients.

In the subsequent chapter, coauthored by Dr. Handel and Dr. Bennett, administrative barriers in planning and implementing gender-specific services are delineated. The authors make it clear that there are enormous inadequacies in our recognition of the specific medical and gynecological needs of chronically mentally ill women. Their observations are of great importance since continuity of care for the chronically mentally ill necessarily includes comprehensiveness (3).

That chronically mentally ill women are often diverted into the criminal justice system is not an irrelevant fact. The criminal involvement of these women, which consists largely of prostitution and petty crime, often results from their difficulty in finding housing and health care. There are data suggesting that women living on the streets and in shelters are more likely than men to have been previously hospitalized for psychiatric disorders, yet there are fewer resources for care for these women (4, 5).

Moreover, "seriously mentally ill women are more likely than men to have direct child care responsibilities and thus this type of disability may have greater impact on a second generation" (6).

Women, furthermore, in their traditional societal role as caretakers, are more likely to bear the responsibility for the care of the chronically mentally ill. There is little public support for family members of the chronically mentally ill, and current changes in patterns of work and family life in our society suggest that working women will bear the additional burden of caring for family members who are mentally ill.

Research and program development for mentally ill women requires that we attend to the changing roles of women in our society and the impact of the changes that are occurring in our health care delivery system. We have not planned for the care of those who are deinstitutionalized or who must leave hospitals prematurely because of insufficient medical insurance coverage. We do not even ask who will care for them when they return to find their place in the community.

Why, then, have we focused on women with chronic mental illness? The reasons may be self-evident. The data presented in this volume indicate that there are large areas of understanding yet to be explored, and many vital needs are yet to be met.

References

1. Lewine RR: Sex differences in schizophrenia: timing or subtypes? Psychol Bull 90:432–444, 1981
2. Chambless DL, Goldstein AJ: Anxieties, agoraphobia and hysteria, in Women and Psychotherapy: An Assessment of Research and Practice. Edited by Brodsky A, Hare-Mustin R. New York, Guilford Press, 1980, pp. 113–134
3. Bachrach LL: Continuity of care for chronic mental patients: a conceptual analysis. Am J Psychiatry 138:1449–1456, 1981
4. Lamb H, Grant R: The mentally ill in an urban county jail. Arch Gen Psychiatry 39:17–22, 1982
5. Stoner MR: The plight of homeless women. Social Services Review 57(4):565–581, 1983
6. Report of the Public Health Service Task Force on Women's Health Issues, in Women's Health, vol II. Washington, DC, US Department of Health and Human Services, 1985